HOW TO START a BUSINESS IN IRIDOLOGY and NUTRITIONAL CONSULTING

Frank Navratil BSc. N.D.

The information contained in this book is for educational purposes only. It is not intended for use in the diagnosis of an individual or health condition except by a qualified health professional. The material is based on the best available research and study by the author at the time of printing and many years of experience in the field of iridology and nutrition. Iridology and nutritional consulting should not be used to replace, but to support a conventional diagnosis. The author is not responsible for any unauthorized use of these methods or for any of the advice given or for any errors that may occur in the text or graphics in this book

How to Start a Business in Iridology and Nutritional Consulting

Published by Return to Health Books

Frank Navratil BSc. N.D.

Purkynova 1246/9

Ricany,

Czech Republic

First Edition

ISBN 978-80-88022-14-5

CONTENTS

PREFACE

Hello and welcome to a new beginning, perhaps, or maybe just a peek into learning about something that may be unfamiliar to you: a career in Iridology and Nutritional Consulting.

My goal here in this book is to share with you my many years of experience as an Iridologist / Clinical Nutritional Consultant and to hopefully clear up any confusion you may have with regards to entering these exciting healing professions. It always pays to know a little about what you are planning to pursue and that is what this book is all about.

I am always very interested to know why you have taken this step. What motivated you to get here at this moment in time? Why are you interested in a career in the healing professions of Iridology and Nutritional Consulting? Perhaps like me you have seen the limitations of modern medicine and have been awakened to a new calling. I personally have to thank my mother who died of cancer many years ago as that event inspired me to follow the path of alternative medicine rather than regular medical school, which I was slated for. What an eye-opener it has been! After seeing more than 20,000 patients over the past 20 years, I can honestly say that I made the right choice. The rewards of a career in the natural healing profession are immeasurable. Natural medicine as opposed to taking drugs is the only method that I believe in. It is the way that nature intended and we must follow the laws of nature in order to truly heal the human body. Iridology and nutrition are one of the most natural healing professions that exist. Iridology, the natural diagnostic instrument and nutrition, the natural healing force and you have a combination that has assisted thousands of people around the world to deal with their health problems.

Starting a successful new career takes a lot of work and clever planning and sometimes a bit of luck. Not only do you have to have the education to perform the work but you also have to have a plan and strategy in place. I sincerely hope that this book will assist you to become the successful professional iridologist or nutritional consultant that I believe you all have the ability to become.

Frank Navratil BSc. N.D.

CHAPTER 1

Why Choose Iridology Or Nutrition As A Career?

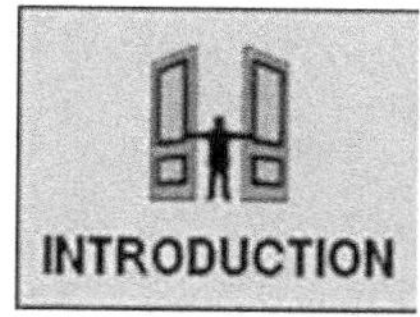

The first chapter of this book examines the advantages of a career in iridology or nutritional consulting. It includes a brief overview of the trends in alternative health care, what iridology and nutritional consulting is all about, the rewards of these healing professions, the important concept of holistic health and what is meant by the iridology-nutrition connection. Included is also an examination of what it takes to enter this profession, barriers that one commonly encounters and attributes for success in this exciting field of natural medicine.

At the end of this chapter you should be able to:

- comprehend some trends that are occurring in alternative health care
- understand the difference between conventional medicine and alternative medicine

- be familiar with some statistics in our modern health care system
- explain what is meant by iridology and nutritional consulting
- explain the concept of holistic health
- understand what is meant by the iridology-nutrition connection
- appreciate what is required to be a professional iridologist or nutritional consultant
- appreciate the rewards of a career in the healing profession
- describe barriers that one often encounters in the alternative healing profession
- list the personal attributes needed for success in the healing profession

Trends in alternative health care

A very practical and logical reason for choosing a career in alternative medicine is that it is a rapidly growing field and there are many reasons why this is currently happening all over the world.

What do we mean by alternative medicine? Well it also comes under the names of complementary medicine, natural medicine, holistic medicine, preventative medicine, and unconventional medicine. Alternative means something different than what conventional medicine offers and scientists generally refer to it as medicine that has not been proved according to scientific methods.

While conventional medicine focuses on destroying illness and disease or neutralizing disease by surgical intervention or chemical intervention (use of drugs), alternative medicine is based on wellness, prevention and maintaining health by strengthening the body both physically, psychologically, spiritually and mentally so that it can fight disease in a natural way. Iridology and nutritional therapy are both natural healing methods and fall under the category of alternative or complementary medicine.

Did you know that up to 90 percent of people around the world have used what we term alternative therapies? Only 10 to 30 percent of people worldwide use conventional medicine and instead use methods that are considered alternative in countries such as the United States. Did you know that in 1998 more than 40 percent of the population of the U.S had used alternative therapy and most had to pay for this care out of their pocket and that this number is growing? Nearly one third of all medical schools in the U.S. including Harvard and Yale now offer courses in alternative medicine. A major national survey on trends in alternative medicine use in the United States was published in the Journal of the the American Medical Association in 1998 and revealed that alternative therapy use increased from 33.8 percent in 1990 to 42.7 percent in 1997. The study showed a 47.3 percent increase in visits to alternative medicine practitioners from 427 million in 1990 to 629 million in 1997, which exceeded total visits to all US primary care physicians! Studies have revealed that 25 to 75 percent of the populations of the United Kingdom, Australia, France, Germany, Israel, Finland, Japan and the Netherlands widely use alternative therapies. In China and India the majority of medical care is provided by traditional providers practicing acupuncture and Ayurveda. In 1993 it was estimated that Australians were spending almost twice as much on complementary medicine than on pharmaceuticals. This means that you are entering a field that is rapidly growing and it's really no wonder. People today expect a lot more from their health care system.

The following trends are influencing this dramatic shift in the traditional health care system in many industrialized nations:

- The population is aging, which is resulting in more chronic health conditions that are currently not adequately being addressed
- Many people with serious health problems such as cancer are using alternative therapies in combination with standard treatment
- People are getting smarter and demanding self-care strategies to prevent illness and to promote wellness
- There is now more of a need for understanding individual differences rather than standard blanket treatment for everyone
- There is greater public awareness of major risk factors that contribute to chronic illness
- In alternative medicine, people can choose whatever they feel works for them and they find this more appealing than traditional health care that dictates what must be done.
- People are taking more control of their own health and not trusting their doctors or conventional medicine practices as much as before
- The attitude of both doctors and common people in western countries is undergoing remarkable change with respect to the outlook towards many alternative therapies that have been practiced for ages in China and India. Many doctors are now recommending alternative therapies to their patients and some studies have shown that up

to 50 percent of doctors in some societies reported using alternative therapies themselves.

- The cost of conventional health care is reaching astronomical levels and many governments cannot afford it anymore

Take a look at this humorous, yet realistic look at Medicine throughout the ages that I picked up from somewhere a long time ago:

MEDICINE THROUGHOUT THE AGES
0001 AD - Here, eat this root.
1000 AD - That root is heathen. Here, say this prayer.
1850 AD - That prayer is superstition. Here, swallow this potion.
1940 AD - That potion is snake oil. Here, swallow this pill.
1985 AD - That pill is ineffective. Here, take this antibiotic.
2000 AD - That antibiotic is dangerous. Here, eat this root.

Well, it certainly seems like we had to take a long unnecessary trip back to where we started. Let's all hope that this positive trend continues but be assured there are still a lot of battles to be won around the world in the sphere of alternative medicine.

Some startling statistics

- In the U.S over 200,000 people die every year of adverse reactions from drugs and another 80,000 die from medical malpractice while only 40,000 die in auto accidents. According to JAMA, doctors kill more people than auto accidents and guns together.
- It was found that in 2003 the pharmaceutical industry did over 182 billion dollars in drug sales worldwide. In contrast to that figure it cost over 183 billion to treat adverse

reactions from all those drugs. By 2020, the industry will top 1 trillion, what will be the cost of adverse reactions then?

- When doctors in Israel were on strike for a month and only very urgent cases were admitted to the hospitals, the death rate dropped by 50 percent. Similar results were found in Bogota, Columbia during a doctor's strike.
- More than 5 percent of all patients admitted to a hospital will get an infection

Hence a crucial need to take a close look at our health system and ask ourselves, is it really helping us or hurting us?

The healing profession of Iridology

Those of you who are new to Iridology or have not yet embarked on taking an iridology course, this section is intended to briefly go over this wonderful method of natural analysis and its application to a career as a healing profession.

What is Iridology?

When people are asked what they look at first when they notice an attractive person, several answers come to mind; some say they notice how a person walks or what a person is wearing. Some notice the perfume or cologne they wear, some take notice of the type of body, or the color and style of hair. However a great proportion of people notice the eyes of a person, for the eyes are often described as the windows to our soul. When we look at people's eyes, we can often determine whether people are lying, whether they are angry or whether they are in love. We often can tell whether people are tired or not feeling well because the eyes will appear dull or lack the usual sparkle when people are not in the best of health. The eye is not only the window to our soul; the eye is a map to our body.

Iridology or iris analysis as it is often called is a method used in alternative medicine to analyze the health status by studying colors, marks and signs in the iris, pupil, and sclera of the eye.

How did iridology start?

Iridology dates back hundreds of years, but the first iris map developed was in the early 1800's by a doctor named Ignatz von Pezcely in Hungary. He is known as the father of iridology. In his childhood it is written that he captured an injured owl in his backyard that had a broken leg. He noticed in one of its eyes that there was a black line but when the leg healed, a white mark appeared where the dark mark was. This incident started a life-long interest and study of iridology. Since then, many scientists, doctors, and health professionals around the world have studied iridology. Iridology is taught in countries like America, Australia, Germany, and Russia, where even modern medicine has begun to take notice.

A career in Iridology

Many medical doctors, healers, natural therapists and laypeople have decided for a career in Iridology. Iridologists are in great demand all over the world as patients are increasingly searching for alternative ways to find the causes of their health problems. Modern medicine unfortunately has its limitations and many diagnostic techniques such as blood tests and x-rays are often painful, invasive and carry with them a certain degree of risk. An Iridology examination is an absolutely safe, non-invasive, painless and reliable method of obtaining information about the health status of an individual and one of the few real methods to view all the body organs and systems as a whole and how they interact with each other. In recent years Iridology and natural medicine have shown unbelievable growth as a career option the world over. The potential is fantastic and Iridology in combination with other natural healing methods such as Nutrition, Homeopathy, Herbal Medicine or vitamin and mineral therapy is providing an effective solution to the growing rate of chronic health problems.

The healing profession of Nutritional Consulting

What is Nutritional Consulting?

Nutritional consulting consists of providing holistic nutritional advice that provides clients with all the nutrients that their individual body requires. It consists of preventative nutrition, nutrition for maintenance of health and nutritional therapy for disease conditions. Providing holistic nutrition takes into account genetic requirements for nutrition as well as nutrients that are required for growth, regeneration from disease, stresses that we impose on our bodies and changes as we age. Nutritional consulting takes into consideration individual needs, as every client is different. The Nutritional consultant recommends foods, vitamins and nutritional supplementation and also devises dietary programs for a variety of health problems and special health conditions.

A career as a Nutritional Consultant

Many medical doctors, healers, natural therapists and laypeople have also decided for a career as a nutritional consultant. Nutritional consultants, like iridologist are also in great demand as patients as more and more research is uncovering nutritional causes of many health problems. Poor nutrition is responsible for the majority of modern health problems that we suffer from today.

In recent years Nutrition and natural medicine have shown unbelievable growth as a career option the world over. The potential is fantastic and Nutrition in combination with other natural healing methods such as Iridology, Homeopathy, Herbal Medicine or vitamin and mineral therapy is also providing an effective solution to the growing rate of chronic health problems.

Holistic Health

We can view holistic health as all the factors that influence our health including nutrition, exercise, emotions, sunlight, job satisfaction, relationships, creativity, nature, and spirituality among many others. This concept is extremely important when working in the healing arts, as even though you may specialize as an iridologist or nutritional consultant, you should always be aware of additional factors that may be contributing to your client's health problems.

The Iridology-Nutrition connection

Your eyes are your connection to your nutritional needs

Earlier on we introduced the subject of Iridology as a natural means of gathering information about our health status by what we see in the iris of our eyes. For years I have been using this science with great success to analyze health problems and to foresee potential health problems. However a natural analytical method is only as good as a healing method that goes along with it. My research with many thousands of patients has revealed some fascinating results between what I have seen in the eyes and the use of advanced nutritional methods. These nutritional methods have been used to strengthen genetic weaknesses and to overcome and prevent disease.

Part of the Iridology course that I have written, is the study of genetic eye constitutions. Each of these genetic eye constitutions has a different combination of common health problems and therefore different nutritional needs. You will find there is a connection between genetic eye constitutions and nutritional needs. I call this the Iridology-Nutrition connection. My new book, *Eat Wise by Reading Your Eyes*, along with my Holistic Nutrition courses on CD-ROM is based on the iridology-nutrition connection.

According to the science of Iridology, our eyes reveal a whole world of information about our genetics and our health status because they are with us every day, every hour, every minute and every second, recording information from messages in our nervous system. These messages show up in our eyes as color pigments and structural signs in the fibers of the iris itself. When we learn to read the signs in our eyes we can understand what body organs or systems are weak so that we can apply the necessary nutritional program.

Applying nutrition to signs seen through Iridology is a safe and effective natural method to deal with chronic problems or to prevent them from ever beginning. Iridology can be used to find solutions for health problems and what organs need to be worked on to enable the body to work more efficiently so that your clients can achieve long-lasting results.

Chinese medicine is based on thousands of years of learning to understand the inner workings of the human body from outside the body. Iridology is no different. The study of Iridology is an exciting and growing science in the field of natural medicine. I believe that Iridology is really the diagnostic method of the future and in combination with nutrition a vital force in the healing process.

Do you have what it takes to be an iridologist or nutritional consultant?

To be a successful and professional iridologist or nutritional consultant you will need:

- Extensive education and knowledge in your field
- Experience
- Confidence
- Willpower
- Dedication
- Determination
- Planning skills
- Business skills
- Marketing skills
- People skills
- Communications skills
- Some tools or equipment

Personal and financial rewards

Everyone has their reasons why they want to enter the healing profession. When we give something of ourselves to others as we do when we assist others with their health problems, we get much back in the form of personal job satisfaction, monetary reimbursement, friendships and trust, and learning through experience. As an iridologist or nutritional consultant in your own business, you have the freedom to work at your time and set appointments to fit your schedule. This allows a lot of flexibility as opposed to a regular job but it also requires more self-motivation and a lot more energy. Most natural therapists who run their own business find that their work does not stop at the end of their last appointment. There is paperwork, planning, marketing, advertising and a host of other odds and ends that take time. In my experience the long days and sometimes nights are worth it in the end. The pride of seeing your own natural therapy business grow and prosper gives you a lot of pride and personal satisfaction that is hard to find in a regular 9 to 5 job.

Although many iridologists and nutritional consultants can earn an excellent living and some may even approach or surpass the salaries of some medical doctors, the majority often do not achieve the success that they expect, because they have not done adequate planning or poorly managed or marketed their business. Money should also not be the only motivator to enter this field. These healing professions require special people; people who have a natural respect for mankind and who have a passion in their work, work that often has the power to change the attitudes and lifestyle habits of their clients. It is an important responsibility that we share in this exciting field. There is no such thing as a perfect job and this applies even to the healing professions. Working with sick people is not an easy thing to do and at times may test your patience and sap your energy levels. But, in my experience, overall the benefits and rewards far outweigh the downside.

Barriers to overcome

So you're fresh out of school and now an educated iridologist or nutritional consultant and the rest is all downhill right? Wrong. Working in the alternative therapies can sometimes be a great challenge. All the great natural therapists of the past had to fight for their right to practice; some were burned at the stake because their methods were seen to be like witchcraft. Well, thank goodness at least that does not threaten us today but you will still encounter barriers.

These barriers can include:

- Laws that may prevent you from practicing in some areas
- Certain restrictions on who you can treat or what diseases you can treat
- Negative clients who do not believe in your methods
- Doctors and those in the medical professions who will put down your methods
- Clients who expect miracles overnight
- Members of your family who will not accept what you are doing

Remember, in order for you to have chosen to enter the field of natural medicine, you already have to be a special person with a different outlook and special attributes. If you believe in what you are doing or planning to do, you will find the strength to overcome these barriers as most of them stem from a lack of understanding of alternative medicine. Over the last 200 years we have been brainwashed into thinking that we cannot assist ourselves without the use of drugs and modern medicine. Most people have forgotten nature's laws including the doctors in our modern health care system. Being an iridologist or nutritional consultant requires strength and determination to overcome these common obstacles. Our role also requires constantly educating our clients so that they see alternative medicine in a new light. In the past I have lectured to many doctors and found that only a very small percentage of them recommend diet for health problems. This still comes as a shock to me as 90 percent of all health problems are often related to what people eat!

Perseverance can change laws and remove restrictions on the practice of natural therapies. Remember it was not that long ago that acupuncture and homeopathy were outlawed. As alternative therapies gain their respected place in our health system, these barriers will diminish, as more and more people will be accepting of these methods. The future looks bright according to those trends but the educational role of the iridologist and nutritional consultant I am sure will still be very important part of our job.

Personal attributes required for success in your iridology or nutritional consulting practice

We spoke before of some attributes that are necessary to be a successful and professional iridologist or nutritional consultant but here is a more exhaustive list.

- High energy levels
- Excellent planning and organizational skills
- Adequate education in iridology and the nutritional sciences
- Understanding of human anatomy and physiology
- Willpower and ability to work on your own
- Knowledge of how to market and advertise your practice
- Empathy and respect for others
- Patience and listening skills
- Confidence and ability to achieve trust and respect
- Desire to expand your knowledge through continuous education
- First -hand experience
- Communication and teaching skills
- Resilience, especially to barriers that often are encountered

If you feel that you have what it takes, let's get on with it and take the first steps to setting up an iridology or nutritional consulting practice. The next chapter will get your started.

Before you go on to the next chapter, however, make sure you read the Chapter Summary and do the Practical and Written assignments as well as test your knowledge through the Self-Test.

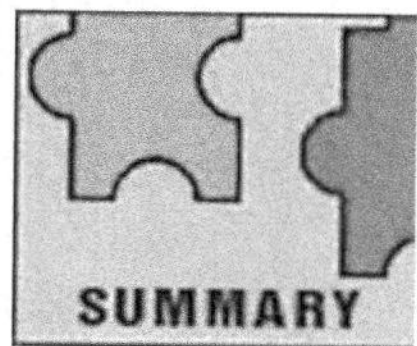

1. Trends in alternative health care show that in most industrialized nations the use of alternative therapies is increasing.
2. In countries such as the United States and Australia, the number of visits to alternative medicine practitioners has surpassed the number of visits to primary care physicians.
3. Reasons for the popularity of alternative medicine include, an aging population and more chronic health problems, greater awareness of self-healing and individual differences, changes in traditional views held by doctors, spiraling costs of our health care system, and lack of trust in our current health system.
4. The medical system and pharmaceutical industry is costing us more lives and money than auto accidents and firearms together.
5. Iridology or iris diagnosis as it is often called is a method used in alternative medicine to analyze the health status by studying colors, marks and signs in the iris, pupil, and sclera of the eye.
6. Nutritional consulting consists of providing holistic nutritional advice that provides clients with all the nutrients that their individual body requires. It consists of preventative nutrition, nutrition for maintenance of health and nutritional therapy for disease conditions.

7. Iridology and nutritional consulting is showing a dramatic growth all over the world.
8. Holistic health includes all the factors that influence our health including nutrition, exercise, emotions, sunlight, job satisfaction, relationships, creativity, nature, and spirituality among many others.
9. There is a connection between genetic eye constitutions studied in iridology and nutritional needs. When we learn to read the signs in our eyes we can understand what body organs or systems are weak so that we can apply the necessary nutritional program. This is called the iridology-nutrition connection.
10. Personal rewards from the healing professions include personal job satisfaction, monetary reimbursement, friendships and trust, and learning through experience.
11. Possible barriers to practicing iridology or nutritional consulting include laws and restrictions, family, clients and doctors who are negative and clients that expect miracles overnight.
12. Some personal attributes for success in this field include: determination, perseverance, confidence, education, empathy, high energy, experience, planning, marketing and business skills, and patience and communication skills.

Please take the time to answer these questions:

1. Describe some the current trends in alternative health care.
2. Discuss some possible reasons for this dramatic shift in our traditional health care system.

3. Describe the meaning of Iridology and what is involved in being an Iridologist.
4. Describe the meaning of a nutritional consultant and what is involved in practicing this healing profession.
5. What is meant by holistic health?
6. What is meant by the iridology-nutrition connection?
7. What are some rewards gained from the healing professions?
8. Describe some barriers that can arise in a career in the alternative therapies.
9. List the important personal attributes required for a successful career in iridology and nutritional consulting.

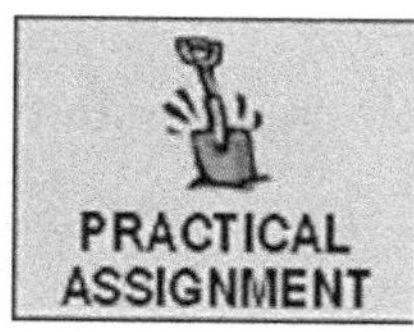

1. Take a look at the geographical area that you live in and analyze some of the trends in alternative medicine. Visit some alternative medicine clinics and ask questions?
2. Find out what are the most common chronic health problems in your area and what most people do to alleviate them.
3. Research to find any iridologists or nutritional consultants in your area and find out what the public opinion of these healing professions is in your area.
4. Investigate the laws and restrictions in your area in regards to practicing iridology and nutritional consulting.

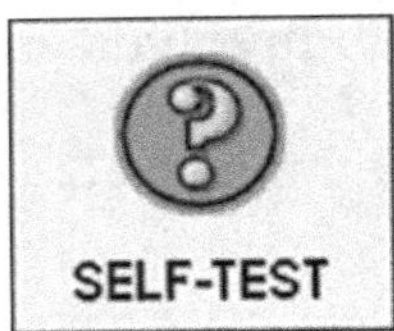

Chapter 1 Self-Test

1. **In most industrialized nations, the trend in utilizing alternative medicine is:**
   a) decreasing
   b) increasing
   c) remaining stable
   d) none of the above

2. **Reasons for a shift in our traditional health-care system may be due to all except:**
   a) an aging population
   b) decrease in chronic health problems
   c) greater awareness of self-healing
   d) lack of trust in present health-care system

3. **Which of these factors cost the most lives in the U.S.?**
   a) traffic accidents
   b) firearms
   c) pharmaceuticals and medical malpractice
   d) none of the above

4. **Iridology is a healing profession that:**
   a) involves analyzing the iris, pupil and sclera
   b) is known only in Hungary
   c) is an invasive form of diagnosis
   d) two of the above

5. **Nutritional consulting is a healing profession that:**
   a) involves only nutrition for disease conditions
   b) does not provide dietary programs
   c) is not in demand around the world
   d) provides holistic nutritional advice

6. **The term "holistic health" means:**
   a) nutritional health only
   b) physical factors only
   c) psychological factors only
   d) all factors that influence health

7. **The Iridology-nutrition connection refers to:**
   a) our eyes being bigger than our stomach
   b) nutrition and how it affects our eyesight
   c) applying nutritional programs by signs seen in Iridology
   d) none of the above

8. **Barriers to practicing iridology or nutritional consulting include:**
   a) laws governing practice of alternative therapies
   b) restrictions on who and what to treat
   c) negative attitudes
   d) all of the above

9. **Personal attributes for success include all except:**
   a) confidence
   b) determination
   c) disrespect
   d) good communication skills

10. **Benefits of working in the healing professions of iridology or nutritional consulting include:**
    a) flexibility in work schedule
    b) personal job satisfaction
    c) both of these healing arts are growing in popularity
    d) all of the above

Answers can be found at the end of the book

CHAPTER 2

Setting Up An Iridology Or Nutritional Consulting Practice

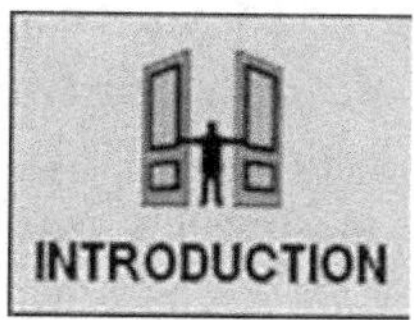

The second chapter of this book examines the first steps in setting up an iridology or nutritional consulting practice. It includes naming your business and developing a logo, determining your mission statement and setting goals and objectives, financial planning, record keeping, locating your business premises and analyzing your competition.

At the end of this chapter you should be able to:

- understand the importance of a business name and company logo
- be familiar with business planning by determining a mission statement, goals and objectives
- be familiar with some statistics in our modern health care system

- make a financial plan related to running an iridology or nutritional consulting practice
- understand what is required for record-keeping
- recognize the importance of analyzing your competition
- appreciate what is required for choosing your business premises

I can appreciate that for those who are not new to starting their own business, this chapter may not be that relevant but for those who will be starting a career and business for the first time, it can often be a daunting process. I will try the best that I know how and from my own experience to share with you some of the basic steps in setting up a natural therapies practice.

Your first start

After you have completed your training in iridology or nutrition, I am sure you are anxious to get started right away, open up shop and start putting what you have learned into practice. Before you rush into it, take some time to take a look at what you are planning to do. Most natural therapy businesses fail within the first year and most of the time it is not because of lack of training but lack of business skills. The sad fact is that most of these failed businesses do not utilize any form of planning.

Your first start requires you to take a broad look at the business you are getting into. It requires that you make some sort of a plan. Among other things your plan should at least contain the following:

- determine your business name and develop a logo
- develop a mission statement and determine goals and objectives
- develop a financial cost analysis for your practice and include insurance
- make a forecast for generated income
- make a short (1 year) and a long-term (3 or more year) plan
- decide what you will require for keeping records of your clients
- analyze your competition
- find a place to run your iridology or nutritional consulting practice

Determining your business name and developing a logo

For many people at first it doesn't seem to matter about what business name you have and many natural therapists will just use their own name, which is fine in most cases. For example: Joe Green, Iridologist. What is important however is that the name of your business identifies your customers or clients with you and your service. From your business name it should immediately tell something to your clients and it is very important, as this company name will stay with you as your business grows and represent what you and your service is all about.

First of all, you should decide what your business is all about or what it will all be about in the future. Will you be just practicing iridology or just nutritional consulting or will you be combining diagnosis with nutritional advice? Will you be selling nutritional supplements and vitamins as well? Will you be teaching or performing seminars? Will you be working domestically or internationally? It is important to make a plan of what you will be doing so that you can come up with a clever business name that will encompass everything that you are all about. Joe Green, Iridologist may suffice in the beginning but as your practice grows, perhaps you may want to open a shop and start selling supplements or products or start a natural therapy school. In that case, maybe a name like Natural Green Health Company may be more appropriate. I chose the name Return to Health International as now my company includes publishing, an iridology and nutrition consulting practice, an international college, as well as natural therapy products.

Not only is your company name important but also is a company logo.

I don't have to explain to you all how important the NIKE logo is to their company and how most people in the world when they see that logo immediately know it belongs to NIKE.

A company logo is another important identification tool that will connect your clients to what your business is all about. Try to come up with a unique idea that will differentiate your natural therapy business from any other one. Try to make it simple. There are many graphical artists that can develop logos from your basic idea. Keep it simple, effective and make sure it communicates your message to your customers. After you develop a logo, use it everywhere you can, on your stationary, on advertising materials, on products, on signs etc.... After effective marketing that can sometimes take many years, your logo may one day be instantly recognizable and just a glance at it will communicate what your business is all about.

As your goal I am sure is to be the most professional and successful iridologist or nutritional consultant, an effective business name and logo are important first steps in starting your business.

Business planning: determining your mission statement, goals and objectives

Every business needs a purpose that says what it is and a vision that describes what it wants to be and this applies even to a natural therapies practice. This purpose and vision come together in the mission statement. A mission statement then becomes the starting point for the development of business goals, and goals are the basis for setting measurable business objectives. It is the first step in your business plan. Every business plan should have a mission statement and goals, and good plans also include objectives. First, let's take a look at what a mission statement is all about.

A Mission Statement

A mission statement is a written declaration of what your business aspires to be. This statement defines the business' reason for being, states why it exists, and clarifies who it serves, as well as expresses what it hopes to achieve in the future. A carefully crafted mission statement accurately describes the business and inspires the people who contribute to its success. It should be broad to encompass everything that you will be doing, short and concise, realistic, easily understood and motivational. When writing your mission statement, ask yourself the following questions:

What business am I really in?

What type of business do I want to be?

What is my target market?

What inspires me?

What is my vision for this business?

What are my main goals to achieve in this business?

Here is an example of the mission statement of Macdonald's restaurants:

> "McDonald's vision is to be the world's best quick service restaurant experience. Being the best means providing outstanding quality, service, cleanliness and value, so that we make every customer in every restaurant smile."

> For example, your mission statement could read:

> Natural Green Health Company will aspire to be the best natural therapy company of its kind in the city of Los Angeles, offering iridology and nutritional consultation service, courses in natural therapy and nutritional supplements for the prevention and treatment of diseases for all members of the family. It will provide the highest quality in service, education and products.

Business Goals

From a planning perspective there is a big problem with a mission statement. It promises a lot but does not say how you intend to deliver on that promise. That is why a business plan also needs goals.

A goal is a statement that clearly describes actions to be taken or tasks to be accomplished. Your business will have a number of goals, each describing a desired future condition toward which efforts are directed. If the goals are accomplished, then the business will be a success.

The purpose of goal setting is to establish a measure for evaluating the success of the business. Goals help keep you focused on success and away from other distractions that drain business resources and accomplish little. The starting point in writing business goals is to ask, "What do I need to do to accomplish my mission." While a mission statement says "why" you are doing what you are doing, business goals say "how" you will do it. Ensure that your business goals state what is to be accomplished as clearly as possible, they should allow for short-term planning and long-term planning. Goals should be specific, challenging but achievable.

Examples of goals that you might have for your iridology or nutritional consulting practice are:

1. Find a business name
2. Develop a business logo
3. Find suitable business premises
4. Attract clientele for iridology and nutritional consultations
5. Have the iridology and nutritional consulting practice pay for itself within 1 year

Business Objectives

While goals define your mission statement, objectives define your goals. An objective is like a sub-goal. It describes exactly a short-term, specific condition that must exist to fulfill a stated goal.

A popular way to remember how to write **SMART** objectives is to remember the letter of the word **SMART**:

Objectives should be **S**pecific, **M**easurable, **A**ction-oriented, **R**ealistic, and **T**ime-oriented.

For example if we go back to number 4 of our goals that we set:

Attract clientele for iridology or nutritional consultations

Some of your objectives could include:

- Put a monthly ad in the local health magazine for the month of September
- Print 1000 flyers and distribute them to all homes in the area by the end of September
- Make a presentation on iridology and nutrition at the local club this month
- Make a note of mentioning my practice to at least 10 friends this week

It is always wise when starting up to come up with a mission statement, set goals and then objectives. In doing so you will have a clear view ahead of what you need to accomplish and how you will go about doing it. A business plan that incorporates these factors ensures that you have the best possible chance of succeeding in your effort to start a professional iridology or nutritional consulting practice.

Developing a financial plan for the running of your practice

Unless you are thinking of starting a charitable organization, one of the reasons you're starting a business is because you think you can make money at it. In order to survive as a business, you have to make money and plan to pay for expenses and operating costs for running the practice. When you develop a business plan, analyzing your expenses is most important. Often it is required when applying for business loans as well as provides a plan to avoid the pitfalls that often occur in failed natural therapy businesses.

If you're like most startup natural therapy businesses, you are probably going to experience at least a short period during which expenses exceed revenue, until of course your client base increases. Without plans for adequate cash reserves, borrowing capacity, or other means of meeting those expenses, a cash shortfall can cause the early demise of your new business. It doesn't matter that the idea behind the business is fundamentally sound; without adequate capital, you won't make it.

Forecasting your sales revenue

One of your first tasks in developing a financial plan is to estimate what you think your total income will be in your first year of business. This is often one of the hardest things to do but it is a vital component of your total business plan. Be realistic and estimate the number of clients you will have on a monthly and yearly basis. Multiply this number by the cost of your service. For example: if you charge 50 dollars for an iridology consultation and you forecast in your first year that you will have 2 clients per day, 10 clients per week and 40 clients per month, your monthly forecasted revenue will be 40 x 50 dollars which equals 2000 dollars. Yearly forecasted revenue (taking 4 weeks holiday) would then be 2000 x 11 or 22,000 dollars.

Calculating your expenses

Let's take a look at some common expenses that arise in setting up and running an iridology or nutritional consulting practice. Most natural therapists start out working out of their home, which can be a good idea until clientele increases and initial expenses are paid off.

Setting up expenses: (if you work out of your home, some of these may not be applicable)

- Office renovations
- Telephones and telephone lines
- Signs
- Lease or rent payments in advance
- Furniture
- Equipment (iridology equipment, computer, fax machine, printer)
- Office supplies
- Nutritional supplements
- Advertising campaign
- Insurance payments

Operating expenses (fixed costs):

- Monthly rent of premises and utilities (heat, light, electricity, water)

- Maintenance
- Telephone bills
- Office supplies
- Nutritional supplements
- Any wages should you employ a secretary or associate
- Advertising
- Insurance for premises and for self
- Postage and freight

It is a good idea to keep costs down as much as possible and this can often be the difference between business success and failure. There will be initial setting up expenses before you even earn any money from your first client, so be prepared to be in the hole for a while. You may need to obtain financing for your initial setup especially if you are planning to set up in an office. By taking a look at your monthly fixed or operating costs, you will get an idea of what your business must earn to break even.

This is just an example: (note: these are just fictitious numbers)

Monthly rent (including heat, light, water)	450 dollars
Maintenance and cleaning	50 dollars
Telephone	50 dollars
Office supplies	75 dollars
Nutritional supplements to keep in stock	200 dollars
Wages (one part-time secretary)	500 dollars
Monthly advertising	50 dollars
Insurance	100 dollars
Postage and freight	50 dollars
Total monthly operating expenses:	**1,525 dollars**

This means that your forecasted sales revenue of 2000 dollars per month based on an estimate of 2 clients a week at 50 dollars for each consultation, you would end up with a profit of 2000-1525 or 475 dollars.

Don't forget to plan not only recurring monthly expenses but also those nasty unexpected expenses that come up (your computer breaks down, needs repair etc.). A financial reserve should always be in place for surprises. One of the ways to ensure the best type of planning is to ensure that you manage your cash flow.

Managing Your Cash Flow

A healthy cash flow is an essential component of any successful business. If you fail to have enough cash to pay your suppliers, creditors, landlords or your employees, you can quickly be out of business. No doubt about it, proper management of your cash flow is a very important step in making your natural therapy business successful.

In its simplest form, cash flow is the movement of money in and out of your business.

Inflows: Inflows are the movement of money into your cash flow. Inflows are most likely from the sale of your goods or consulting services to your customers.

Outflows: Outflows are the movement of money out of your business. Outflows are generally the result of paying expenses. If your business involves reselling goods such as nutritional supplements then your largest outflow is most likely to be for the purchase of inventory.

I don't want to get into too much detail (If you are like me, most natural therapists despise anything to do with financial matters) but it is very important to analyze your cash flow situation. Ensuring that your inflows (income generated from sales of your products or consulting service) are maximized and delaying some of your outflows (perhaps you can negotiate paying for vitamin supplements a month or two after delivery), will optimize your cash flow situation and allow for financial reserves.

Long-range financial forecasts

After constructing a one-year forecast, you should develop a more detailed long-range or three-year forecast to assist in planning the business. Ensure that you include the set-up costs, monthly fixed costs of operating the business as well as forecasted revenue for the 3 years. Determine if you will profit from the business after 3 years. This is a useful tool to determine if you need to find ways to reduce expenses or increase revenues.

Record-Keeping

I am sure that unless you aspire to be an accountant, record keeping is not on the top of your list in priorities. It is however, important to keep some records in an iridology or nutritional consulting business. Some of these records include:

- Client records
- Iridology or nutritional consultation reports
- Accounting records
- Inventory records

Client Records

It is important to keep a client database so that you have accurate contact details on each. You may need to send them information from time to time or to contact them. There are many computer software programs including iridology software that includes a client database along with the ability to store iridology reports. Having the client's details and consultations reports ready at hand is very important should the client require assistance.

Iridology or nutritional consultation Records

This area will be discussed in more detail in a later module but keeping records of your consultation reports and recommendations is vital. There are times when clients lose their reports and a copy of these reports is essential to have when clients come for their next appointment. It is also a document that you must have in the event of any legal action or lawsuits that could arise as a result of your recommendations. Otherwise you would have no proof of what you recommended in terms of nutrition or otherwise for your client.

Accounting Records

Various financial records are often required. See you accountant for details pertaining to your type of business.

Inventory Records

If you are selling goods like nutritional supplements, you will need to have inventory records of what you have in stock and what has been sold.

Analyzing your competition

This is often an overlooked consideration when starting a new business. By analyzing your competition, you can, not only find out a wealth of information on the business climate in general but also how to go about doing what you plan to do. Seeing that there is competition in the same area of business as you are, indicates that there is a market for your products or service out there. It may also assist you in what location you should set up your own consulting service. Don't panic if there is an iridologist or nutritional consultant nearby where you are located. Attracting clients depends not on the number of you out there but the quality and professionalism of your services. Assessing the competition, the services that they provide and their costs can assist you to formulate your own strategies so that you can achieve success and find ways to improve on the benefits that they already have. Depending on where you are in the world, there is always some competition lurking around somewhere and if there isn't there soon will. Never bad-mouth your competition, as this only advertises your insecurity and will detract clients. Be confident in your abilities and services and strive to perform the best service possible. In the field of iridology and nutrition there is just so much business out there at the moment and so many clients out there who need such a service, that I believe in most areas of the world it will take many, many years for the industry to become saturated.

Choosing your business premises

When starting your own iridology or nutritional consulting practice there are basically three main options that are open in regards to business premises:

1. Work out of your own home
2. Share an office
3. Rent your own office

Working out of your own home

This option is obviously the most economical and often the starting point for many natural therapists who enter the field. In most cases a portion of the expenses on your home can be written off as expenses and you do not incur extra expenses in the form of rent or utilities. If you are unsure or do not have adequate capital, I would recommend you to start in this way until you have built up a clientele and have adequate financial resources. Another option is that you can also offer an mobile service where you can go to your client's home and offer your consultation services in their premises.

Sharing an office

Many natural therapists who rent their own office are often looking for an associate to rent a room or share an office with them. Many alternative therapy clinics have a central secretary that handles incoming calls and messages for many natural therapists working at the same office. This reduces the operating cost per therapist as office equipment like computers and copiers are shared and expenses are shared. This option provides professional surroundings without the heavy costs that can be incurred having your own office. It also can offer more flexibility in the event that you want to leave the premises and change locations.

Renting your own office for your practice

This option is the most costly as the iridologist or nutritional consultant is responsible for all expenses, rent and utilities. It has the advantage that you can operate your clinic as you wish but with a much higher price to pay. It is harder to leave the premises especially after signing long-term leases.

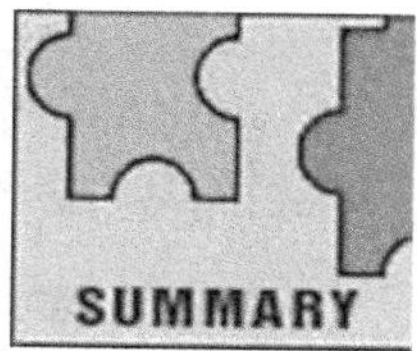

1. A business name and logo should reflect your business and be easily recognizable.
2. A mission statement is a written declaration of what your business aspires to be. This statement defines the business' reason for being, states why it exists, and clarifies who it serves, as well as expresses what it hopes to achieve in the future.
3. A goal is a statement that clearly describes actions to be taken or tasks to be accomplished. Your business will have a number of goals, each describing a desired future condition toward which efforts are directed. If the goals are accomplished, then the business will be a success.
4. An objective is like a sub-goal. It describes exactly a short-term, specific condition that must exist to fulfill a stated goal. Objectives should be **S**pecific, **M**easurable, **A**ction-oriented, **R**ealistic, and **T**ime-oriented.
5. Developing a financial plan for your practice involves forecasting your short-term and long-term sales revenue, calculating expenses and managing your cash flow.
6. Record keeping is an important component on a consulting practice. Client records, consultation records, accounting records and inventory records are some that the iridologist or nutritional consultant should be familiar with.
7. Analyzing your competition is a useful way to gather information and to understand the market and what role your business will play.

8. When you are deciding on business premises you have the choice of working out of your own home, sharing an office of clinic or opening up your own. Each one has its advantages and disadvantages.

Please take the time to answer these questions:

1. Why is a business name and logo important for an iridology or nutritional consulting practice?
2. What is a mission statement?
3. What is the difference between a goal and an objective?
4. What are the components of a financial business plan?
5. Describe some types of records that an iridologist or nutritional consultant should be familiar with.
6. Describe the advantages and disadvantages of the three main options of business premises available to the iridologist or nutritional consultant.

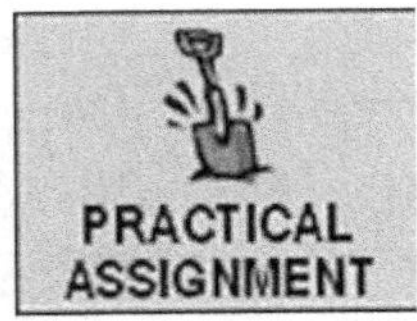

1. Come up with your own business name and try to come up with some ideas for a logo.
2. Write down the mission statement for your business.
3. Write down the major goals for your business.

4. Write down clear and achievable objectives for your first month in business.
5. Take the time to construct a financial plan, which include short and long-term plans. Write down a list of your anticipated expenses and make a forecast for projected revenue. Write down any ideas that will maximize your cash flow.
6. Decide what the best option for you is in terms of business premises.
7. Examine the competition in your area.

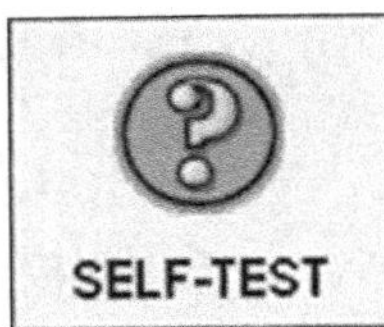

Chapter 2 Self-Test

1. **A business name and logo should be:**
   a) relatively simple
   b) easily recognizable
   c) unique
   d) all of the above

2. **A mission statement:**
   a) states the purpose of the business
   b) should not motivate employees
   c) should state whom the business serves
   d) two of the above

3. **Business goals should be all except:**
   a) challenging
   b) achievable
   c) general
   d) specific

4. **Business objectives should be:**
   a) realistic
   b) measurable
   c) time-oriented
   d) all of the above

   An effective financial plan includes all but:
   a) forecasting sales revenue
   b) stating your mission
   c) calculating expenses
   d) analyzing cash flow

5. **Managing cash flow involves:**
   a) maximizing inflows
   b) maximizing outflows
   c) minimizing outflows
   d) two of the above

6. **Consultation records are important for all except:**
   a) legal protection
   b) consulting with return clients
   c) recording stock
   d) to provide a record of your recommendations

7. **Analyzing the competition allows one to:**
   a) assess the general business climate
   b) better choose a business location
   c) gather important information about the market
   d) all of the above

8. **The least expensive option when considering business premises is:**
   a) sharing an office
   b) renting your own office
   c) working out of your own home
   d) none of the above

9. **When deciding to start your own business it is most important to:**
   a) implement effective planning
   b) determine your costs and forecast revenue
   c) state what your goals and mission are
   d) all of the above

Answers can be found at the end of the book

CHAPTER 3

Equipment Recommended For Your Iridology Or Nutritional Consulting Practice

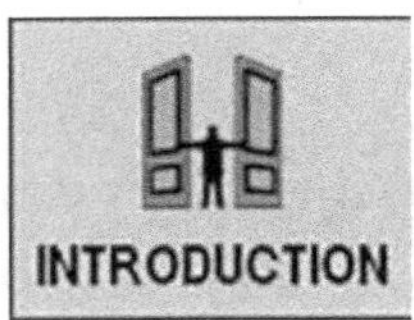

The third chapter of this course examines some equipment that is recommended to run a professional iridology or nutritional consulting practice. It includes an explanation of a variety of tools that the iridologist or nutritional consultant uses in the course of daily practice. A discussion of professional iridology equipment and nutritional products is also included.

At the end of this module the student should be able to:

- be familiar with various tools that the iridologist or nutritional consultant uses in daily practice
- to be aware of what professional iridology equipment is available
- appreciate the role of nutritional products

Tools used by an iridologist

Iridology charts

An Iridology chart is one of the first tools that an iridologist uses daily. Whether it is desk-sized or a wall chart or incorporated into software programs, it assists in finding the locations of body organs as they are reflected in the iris of the eyes. Ignatz von Peczely, a Hungarian homeopathic doctor developed the first iridology chart in the late 1800's. Since then, a variety of different charts or maps of the iris have evolved into what exists in the world today. It must be remembered that an iridology chart is only a guide and an experienced iridologist takes in all signs and discoloration seen in the iris, pupil and sclera along with information from the iridology chart in order to make a more accurate analysis of the client's health status. Most iridology charts show the right and left iris and the various zones and body organ sectors. An iridologist who looks into the client's eyes through a microscope or magnifying lens relies on the iridology chart as a guide to determine what body organs are weak. For those iridologists who use advanced methods such as iridology reporting software, using this software the iridologist can overlay an iridology chart directly over the image of the iris. This allows a much more efficient and accurate method of identifying weak body organs. This software will be discussed in more detail below. A variety of iridology charts like the one below are available at Return to Health International. Just check our web site: www.irisdiagnosis.org for more information.

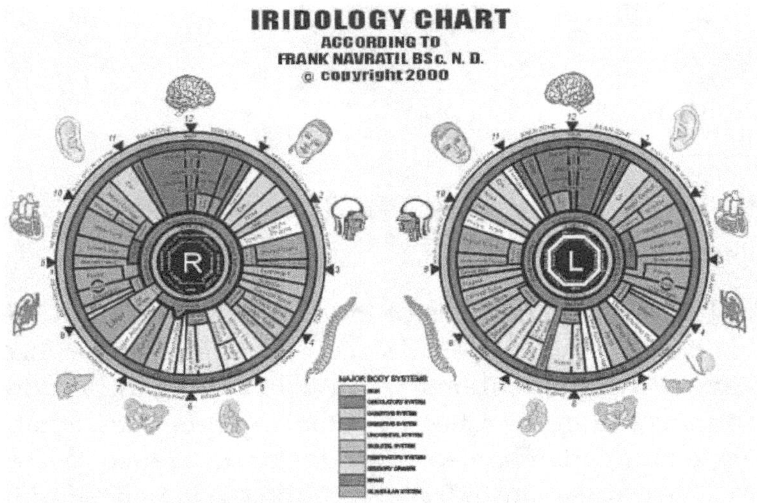

www.irisdiagnosis.org

Iridology flashcards and posters

The beginning iridologist, before gaining experience in the field often must refer to books or manuals for signs and markings seen in the eyes. Useful tools are iridology flashcards that show images of real irises with arrows pointing to the major signs with explanations of what they mean. Not only is this a useful tool for the iridologist but is also an excellent way to show and explain signs to clients. Wall charts of iridology signs and explanations are also available.

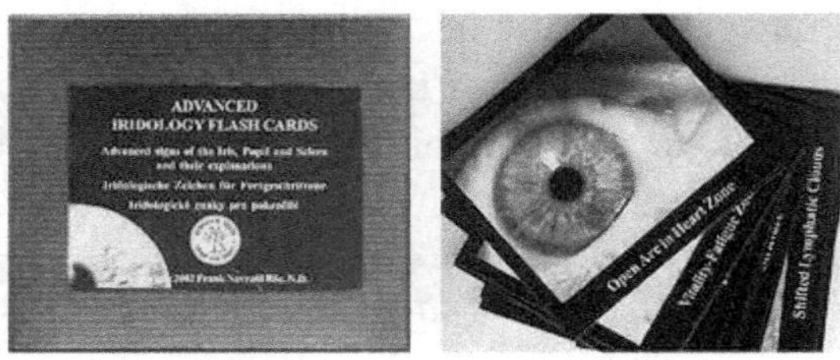

www.irisdiagnosis.org

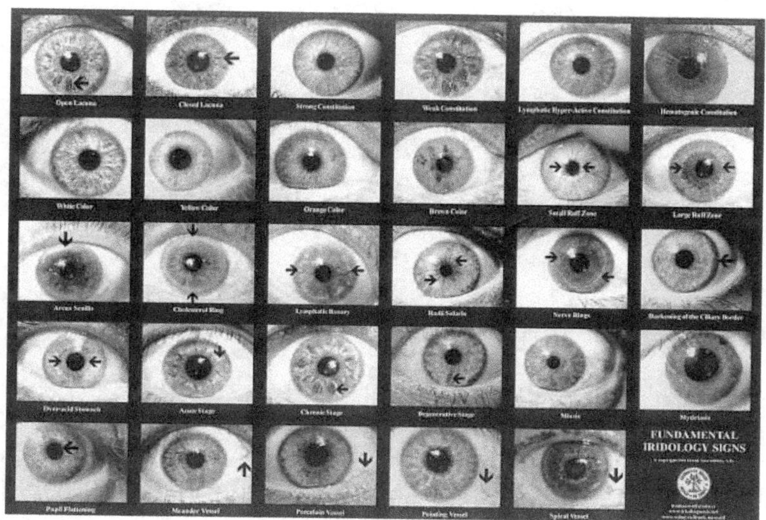

www.irisdiagnosis.org

Magnifying lenses

An economical way to view the human iris is through a magnifying lens. A magnification power of 8-10X is suitable for excellent viewing of the iris and the lens should be combined with a light source. The light source should ideally be aimed at right angles to the iris, which unfortunately most combination magnifying lenses and lights are not equipped to provide this. For this reason, I developed the Iris Mistr® magnifying lens, specifically for the use of iridology, which allows the iridologist to adjust the angle of the lens and light source to their needs. The disadvantage with any magnifying lens is that the client must hold their eyes open for longer periods, which can cause some discomfort for some people. However, it is an excellent way to see true colors and depth of structure which is a reason why I still have it in my practice at all times even though I use a digital iriscope camera system.

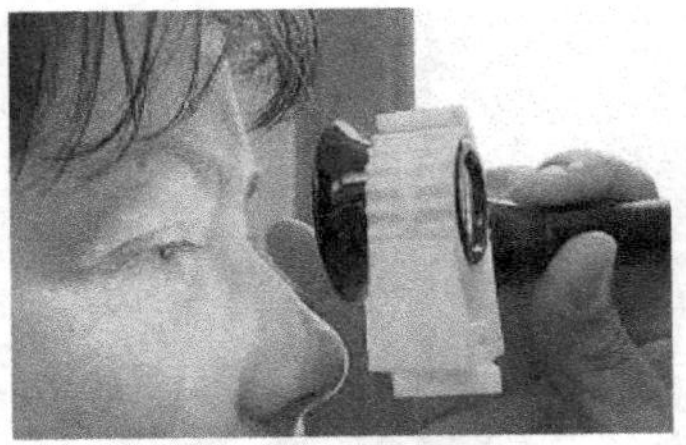

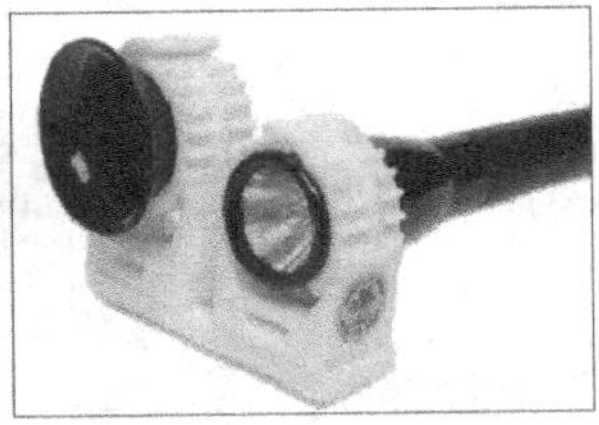

www.irisdiagnosis.org

Iridology resource books and iridology courses

The iridologist should have a good selection of iridology books for reference. Many have been written around the world and it is a very good idea to understand and study all types of methods to get a broad understanding of the subject of iridology. It is also highly recommended to take some iridology courses or classes. If you are interested in some books or courses on iridology, I recommend my books, Iridology: For Your Eyes Only, and Eat Wise by Reading Your Eyes as well as the associated For Your Eyes Only iridology courses. More detailed information on the courses can be found in Chapter 9.

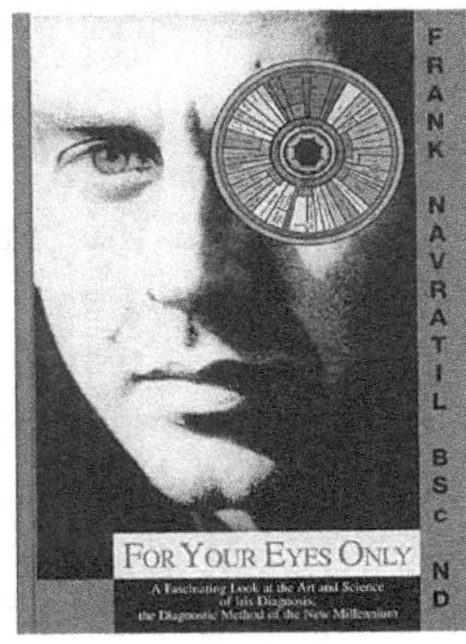

Iridology: For Your Eyes Only
www.irisdiagnosis.org

Iridology software resources

A professional iridologist not only has reference books and texts that are available but for quick reference on the computer, there are many software resources that are available.

In a busy iridology practice or for learning advanced iridology techniques, it pays to have an extensive encyclopedia of iridology at your fingertips. Iridology software resources include Iridology signs seen in the iris, pupil and sclera, Genetic Eye Constitutions, Iris Case Studies and special resources that specialize in Brown-Eye Iridology. More information on the software resources can be found in Chapter 9.

Iriscopes and iridology analysis, scanning and reporting software

Basic hand-held iriscope cameras

Besides the simple magnifying lens there are other ways to view the human iris. Basic hand-held iriscope cameras are available that plug into the USB port of your computer and include internal lights. The iris can be viewed on the computer and images can be captured digitally. For the iridologist they have the advantage of less cost. However, they have the disadvantage that the clients head is not always held in a straight position and capturing the image can be sometimes awkward.

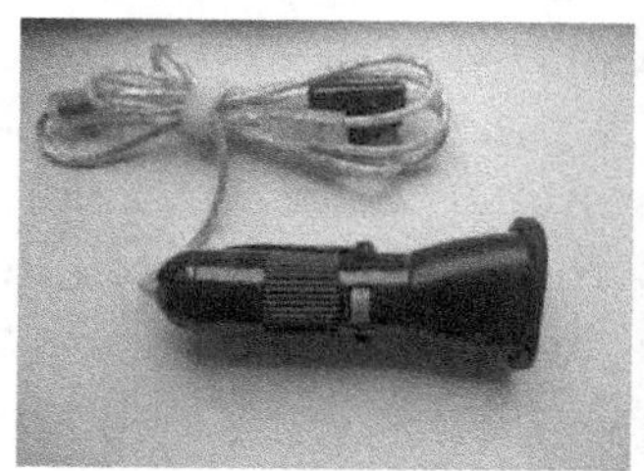
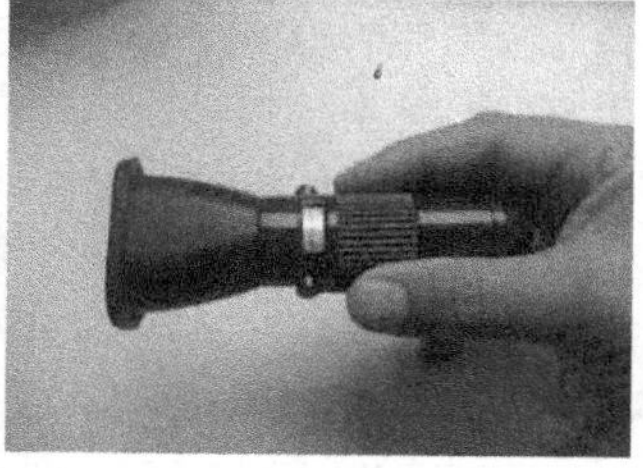

Basic Hand-held iriscope camera
www.irisdiagnosis.org

Professional Digital iriscope cameras

The digital age has brought about a whole range of digital cameras and along with digital cameras came the digital iriscope. With most digital cameras on their own there is a difficulty with capturing a quality iris image and usually special lighting and lenses must be used. The other disadvantage with just a plain digital camera is that the images usually cannot be viewed on the computer live while photographing the irises, but on a small screen at the back of the camera, which can sometimes be difficult to focus in on. Nevertheless they have the ability to capture high-resolution images.

I have found that it is very important to have the camera and client in a stable position to capture a quality iris image. For this reason, another tool for the iridologist that has been developed in combination with the digital camera is the iriscope camera stand with chin and forehead rest. The chin rest allows the client's chin and forehead to be held in a stable position while photographing. Also, xyz movement of the camera is necessary so that you can move the camera up and down to the level of the eye, from side to side to see the left and right iris, and forward and back so that you can focus in on the image.

Special digital cameras with stands that interfaces with your computer are now available that allows you to view the human iris on the screen of your computer and take a snapshot when you have it in focus. The camera is mounted on a movable base and tripod system that allows for xyz movement and includes a chin rest and forehead support for the client. Images are saved directly into your computer where they can be used for analysis through special iridology reporting software. If you are serious about iridology as a career, I sincerely recommend that you get yourself a digital camera with a stand and chin rest along with analysis software. It will increase your ability to analyze the iris more accurately and will save you time. I have developed the Professional Iriscope Camera below which is a cost-effective method that utilizes a stand with a chin rest.

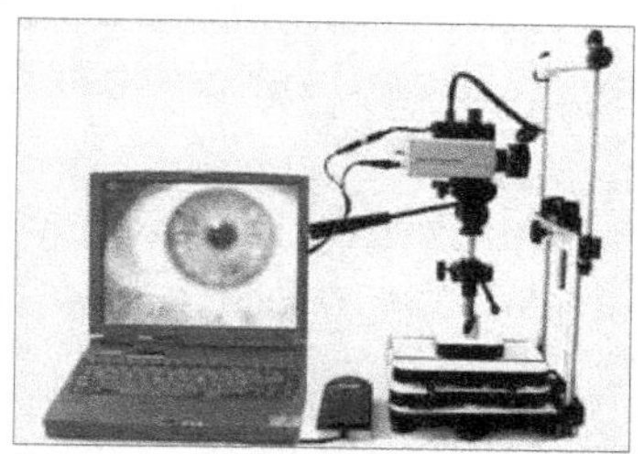

Professional Iriscope camera system
www.irisdiagnosis.org

Iridology analysis and reporting software

While a digital iriscope camera has the function of capturing an image of the iris, iridology analysis and reporting software is another excellent tool that is often used by the professional iridologist in combination with a digital iriscope camera.

What does Iridology analysis and reporting software offer?

- the ability to overlay a right and left iridology chart directly on any iris image
- the ability to automatically scan the iris image and see graphical results of color intensity for every sector of the iris in seconds. At a glance you can see which organ sectors of the iris are degenerative, chronic, sub-acute or acute.
- the ability to store client iris records along with personal information, treatments, etc.

- the ability to label the iris image with text or arrows
- the ability to zoom into any area of the iris image
- the ability to design custom templates for any sector of the iris that will automatically show up in your iridology report with just a click of your mouse on any sector of the iris. These will allow you the flexibility to add any information you wish including treatments for any sector of the iris
- the ability to automatically insert your iris images into professional iridology reports and print them out with ease.
- the ability to save you time in developing professional iridology reports for your clients

For more information on tools for iridology, software resources, digital camera systems and iridology reporting software, please see our web site: www.irisdiagnosis.org

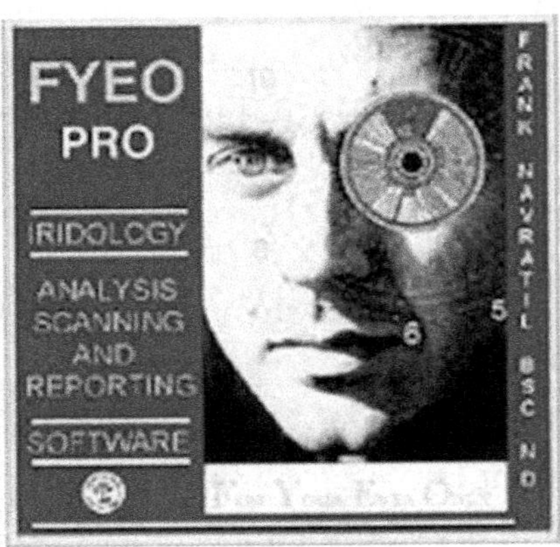

FYEO PRO Iridology analysis, scanning and reporting software program
www.irisdiagnosis.org

Tools used by a nutritional consultant

Nutrition books and nutrition courses

A host of books have been written on the subject of nutrition. It is important for the nutritional consultant to be up-to-date on current issues in nutrition. Therefore good reference material that includes food information, diets, food additives, etc is a must for any nutritional consultant. It is also highly recommended to take some nutrition courses or classes. If you are interested in some books or courses on nutrition, I recommend my book, Eat Wise by Reading Your Eyes, which is a general overview of human nutrition as well as its connection to iridology and the associated Holistic Nutrition courses. More detailed information on the courses and resources can be found in Chapter 9.

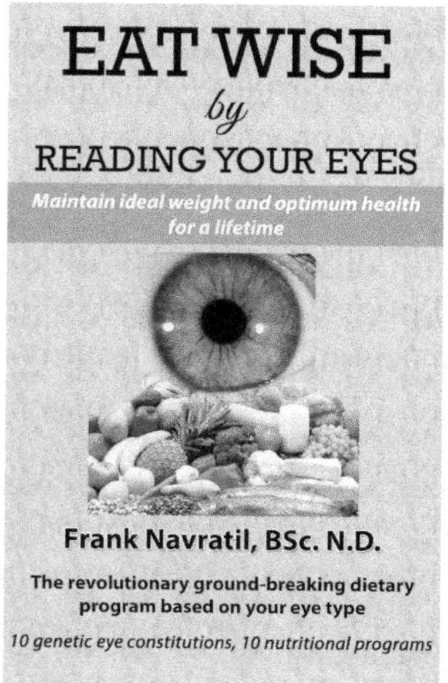

Eat Wise by Reading Your Eyes
www.irisdiagnosis.org

Nutritional software resources

A professional nutritional consultant not only has reference books and texts that are available but for quick reference on the computer, there are also software resources that are available.

It is important to be able to access information on foods, additives, and diets etc. quickly. Nutrition software resources include nutrient information that retrieves at the touch of your fingertips, information of foods, supplements, herbs, vitamins, minerals, additives, and nutrients for diseases. More information on nutrition software resources can be found in Chapter 9.

Nutritional vitamins and supplements

A nutritional consultant usually not only recommends a dietary regime but often supplies nutritional supplements for their clients. In many cases this forms a large percentage of their income in their practice. Today there are so many different brands that are available that include anything from vitamins and minerals to herbs and concentrated nutrients. It is important to have a good knowledge in nutritional therapy and of toxic effects of over-dosage if you plan to offer these to your clients, as well as quality suppliers that offer the highest quality of natural products.

There are other tools that the nutritional consultant may find advantageous such as skinfold calipers for measuring percentage of fat, live blood analysis, urine tests, blood tests, and other specialized equipment that is beyond the scope of this course and in many cases involves medical expertise. Iridology is an excellent non-invasive diagnostic tool for the nutritional consultant to gain more information on the health status of the client so that specific nutritional programs can be developed to suit individual needs.

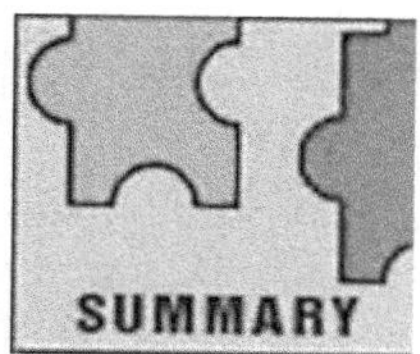

1. One of the most useful tools for the iridologist is an iridology chart that allows identification of body organ sectors in the right and left iris.
2. Iridology flashcards or wall charts showing Iridology signs are useful to explain what you have found to your clients.
3. An economical tool for the iridologist is the magnifying lens. Ensure that it has a light source that is directed at right angles to the eye and a 8-10x magnification lens.
4. Iridology reference books, courses and resources give the professional iridologist a wide resource of easily accessible information about iridology.
5. Basic and Professional iriscope cameras allow digital capture of the iris for analysis.
6. Iridology analysis and reporting software allows you to overlay charts on the iris, to scan the iris for color intensity and to assist in producing professional iridology reports.
7. Nutrition reference books, courses and software resources give the professional nutritional consultant a wide resource of easily accessible information about nutrition and its role in prevention and treatment of disease.
8. A nutritional consultant will often recommend or supply supplements for their clients. It is important to have a good knowledge of the effects of supplements and training in nutritional therapy.

Please take the time to answer these questions:

1. What is an iridology chart?
2. How can iridology flashcards or wall charts assist the iridologist?
3. What is the most economical way to view the human iris?
4. Name some resources that are available for the iridologist.
5. What is a digital iriscope camera? Name and explain some of its components.
6. What does iridology analysis and reporting software allow the iridologist to do?
7. Name some resources that the nutritional consultant has at his or her disposal.
8. What is important about recommending nutritional supplements?

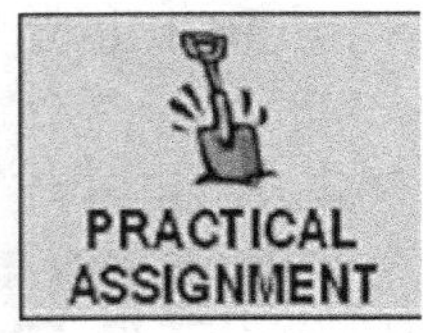

1. Ensure that you have adequate training in iridology or nutrition or take a course.
2. Get yourself an iridology chart as well as an iridology-magnifying lens

3. Start acquiring some iridology resources in the form of books, reference texts, and software resources to improve your knowledge in iridology.
4. If you plan to seriously work as an iridologist and have the budget, look into purchasing a digital iriscope camera and iridology reporting software that will suit your needs.
5. If you plan to be a nutritional consultant, acquire as many books on nutrition and resources as possible to improve your knowledge in nutrition.
6. Investigate the opportunities in prescribing nutritional supplements. Find a quality supplier.

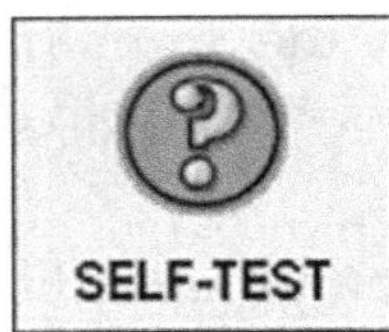

Chapter 3 Self-Test

1. **An iridology chart shows:**
   a) diseases in the body
   b) body organs as they are reflected in the iris
   c) symptoms in the body
   d) none of the above

2. **An iridologist can use what tools:**
   a) iriscope
   b) iridology software
   c) magnifying lens
   d) all of the above

3. **The light source of a magnifying lens should ideally be directed:**
   a) directly on the eye
   b) at right angles to the eye
   c) at a forty-five degree angle to the eye
   d) none of the above

4. **The benefits of magnifying lenses include:**
   a) you cannot see the eye very clearly
   b) they work best with a light source
   c) you can see the eye very clearly
   d) two of the above

5. **Iriscopes include all except:**
   a) basic cameras
   b) professional cameras with stands
   c) digital cameras
   d) iridology reporting software

6. **Components of a digital iriscope system include all except:**
   a) a digital camera
   b) xyz movement
   c) self-analysis mirror
   d) a chin stand and forehead support

7. **A nutritional consultant can use all of these tools:**
   a) nutrition books
   b) nutrition software resources
   c) nutritional supplements
   d) all of the above

8. **Nutritional software resources can:**
   a) allow a quick way to find information on foods
   b) allow a quick way to find information on supplements
   c) calculate blood analysis
   d) two of the above

9. **When recommending nutritional supplements it is important to:**
   a) have training in nutritional therapy
   b) have an understanding of toxic effects of over-dosage
   c) have a quality supplier
   d) all of the above

10. **Tools used by an iridologist or nutritional consultant:**
    a) do not take the place of knowledge and experience in the field
    b) are only effective in the hands of an experienced practitioner
    c) are never required
    d) two of the above

Answers can be found at the end of the book

CHAPTER 4

Marketing Your Iridology Or Nutritional Consulting Practice

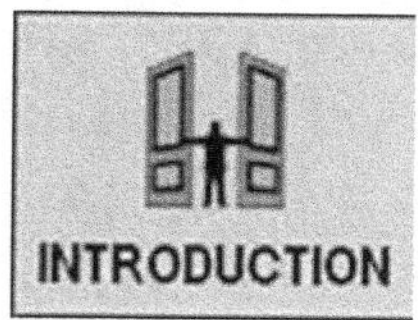

The fourth chapter of this book examines the use of marketing techniques to promote your iridology or nutritional consulting practice. It includes basic marketing research techniques, development of your service, promotion strategies and pricing. Topics discussed also include finding the right location for your premises, learning from your competition and building a solid client base.

At the end of this chapter you should be able to:

- be familiar with various marketing research techniques
- able to identify what your service to your clients will be
- understand various methods used to promote a practice
- know how to effectively price your service
- appreciate the importance of location of your premises
- understand what you can learn from your competition
- identify ways to build a solid client base

How to use basic marketing research when starting an iridology or nutritional consulting practice

Marketing Research

What does the word marketing research really mean? Marketing research is simply the study of markets or groups of people that you would like to sell your iridology or nutritional consulting service to. In other words, it is learning about your customers or clients. Who are they? What do they want or need? These are the types of questions you will need to ask yourself when you begin any marketing research. It is very useful to do some preliminary research before you set up your iridology or nutritional consulting practice.

Common characteristics of clients:

All clients generally have these essential characteristics:

They have a particular need. Your clients have a need for preventative health, for solving their particular health problem or a need for information about their health.

They have the power to make a decision. **The client** has the actual authority to say "yes" or "no" to obtain your iridology or nutritional consulting service.

They have enough money to obtain your service. Make sure that just because a client is interested in an iridology or nutritional consultation, does not mean that they have enough money to obtain it.

They have easy access to your service. **It is very important that your practice is accessible to the clients that you want to target.**

When performing marketing research follow the following steps:

Step 1

Answer the following questions:
What need does my service satisfy?
Who needs and can afford what I am offering?
Who has the authority to say "yes" to the service I am offering?
How accessible is my service to my customers?

Your answers to these questions will form the foundation of your marketing research.

Step 2

Visualize your "ideal" client who will come in for an iridology or nutritional consultation

Utilize demographics

Demographics is the study of the characteristics of a group of people that includes factors like age, income level, sex, family status, lifestyle habits, health status etc.

One of the most effective ways to learn about your client in your geographical area is to visualize what they may actually be like. Are they predominantly young or old or both? What do they do? What health problems do they have? What are they interested in? Once you have a clear picture of what your potential client looks like, try to imagine what their priorities might be in relation to your service. For example, some people may make an appointment for an iridology or nutritional consultation if it is conveniently located and will pay more for this service. Others may find it more convenient to buy their supplements from you than from the local health store. It is important to get into the head of your clients. Try to think like they think. Anticipate what their needs will be. Ensure that your iridology or nutritional consulting service will give them what they want.

Step 3

Determine your primary and secondary markets

Now that you have visualized your clients and gathered demographic information about them, you can take the next step. Although many types of people may be interested in your service, you need to narrow it down and determine who the majority of your customers will be. You can call this group your **primary market**. Your primary market will often have similar characteristics, needs, income levels, lifestyle habits, health problems, etc. This group will provide the majority of business for your practice. Your **secondary market** will consist of the next highest purchasing group with similar characteristics and needs.

For example:

Let's go back to our earlier example from Module 2, and our fictitious Natural Green Health Company.

Your primary market may be for example: all female clients in the age group between 40 and 60, who are relatively sedentary and in the middle class income group.

Your secondary market may be: all females under 40 and males and children.

Step 4

Gather information directly from the source

Once you have done all your homework and have a good idea of who your primary customers are, the best thing you can do is go directly to the source. You can gather information about your primary market in the following ways:

1. **Ask your primary target group some questions**. The greatest benefit to you is that you will learn a lot about the group you are studying including common trends, emotional motivators, and general likes and dislikes of your primary market. You will find out if your iridology or nutritional consulting service would be a benefit to these people and what they are looking for in a natural therapy service.
2. **Conduct a written survey**. The other way is to perform a survey which people can fill out and answer questions. This method has the benefit that it takes less time but it needs to be made up of thoughtful questions that will provide the information that you are looking for.

Marketing research is a critical step in the business planning process, which many small natural therapy practices tend to ignore. It will assist you in making decisions in the future and will prevent you from falling into the habit of developing a service that does not satisfy the needs of your primary market. Remember get into the heads of your clients and you will develop the best possible iridology or nutritional consulting service in your area.

Most marketing that is taught comes in the form of the 4 P's, product, promotion, price and place. The next section will cover all these marketing areas.

How to develop your iridology or nutritional consulting service

The first of these essential P's is **PRODUCT.** As iridologists or nutritional consultants, your product is really your service that you offer. You offer an iridology consultation or a nutritional consultation for your clients. It is important to clarify exactly what your service is. For example, you need to decide how you will offer your service. Will your consultation consist of giving your clients a written iridology or nutrition report or verbal advice or a combination of both? Will you offer nutritional supplements or other health products? How long will the consultation take? Will there be any follow-up consultation? What type of health conditions will you be specializing in? or will you be open for any type of health problem or condition? It is important for you to really clarify what you will actually be offering as your Product or service.

How to promote your iridology or nutritional consulting practice

The second "P" in your marketing strategy is **PROMOTION.** This is a wide-open area and consists of any method that will make your target market aware of your service.

Let's start with some ways that are effective:

1. **Advertising**

   In order for you to reach your target market, especially your primary market, you need to advertise and make your clients aware of the service that you are offering. There are many types of advertising; there is advertising in newspapers, in health magazines, through flyers and posters, web sites, radio and TV. Which one do you choose? Well unless you have an unlimited budget which most of us don't, television is usually out of the question, unless you can get a free spot on a health talk show as a guest. Local radio may be another form of advertising that can be effective, especially if you can book yourself as an expert in your field.

   First of all, try to get as much free publicity and advertising as you can. Iridology and Nutrition are very interesting topics and many magazines will welcome your articles on your field of expertise. Contact local health or alternative health magazines and try to write an interesting article for them. One of the first things that started my career was an article that I wrote about iridology for a health magazine. The day after the magazine was released, I received over 30 telephone calls a day for two weeks. Health and alternative medicine are sought after current topics in today's society and there is so much about them that is constantly being written. I have subsequently written articles and series of articles in well over 100 magazine issues since then.

Probably the best method of advertising and promotion is word of mouth. A satisfied client will tell others and in this way your practice will grow. The beginnings are always difficult but if you believe in what you are doing and are good at what you do and can offer your clients what they need, then you cannot help but succeed. I cannot count the amount of times that a woman comes to me for an iridology consultation, then drags her husband the next time and then the whole family comes. This spreads to neighbors, other relatives, and friends and soon you are running a very busy practice. As I mentioned in the first module, alternative health is a rapidly growing field and almost everyone needs at some point in their lives some form of advice on their health. You just have to convince them that you are the one they need.

Get your iridology or nutritional consultation service on the Internet. Today it is essential that you have a web site. So many clients will find you that way. Ensure that your site is easy to understand, professional, clear and concise. Ensure that you also have an email address as many use this form of communication today.

Another effective, yet relatively economical way to advertise is to produce a flyer. You can easily produce a flyer on your iridology or nutritional consulting service and hand it out to existing or potential clients. I find that flyers are a much better tool than just business cards. Make your flyer easy to read and interesting, that which will capture the attention of your clients. Flyers can be distributed through the postal service, at health conventions or trade shows, or at health stores.

Placing ads in the classified health sections of newspapers or health magazines is also a relatively inexpensive way to attract clients. Again, you will have to experiment which local publications offer the best results.

2. **Local trade shows and conferences**
   Setting up your own booth at a trade show that specializes in health or alternative medicine is an excellent way to promote your practice and target people who are interested in your field. It usually involves a bit more investment but it has the advantage that a large quantity of visitors who attend will be the ones that you want to target.

3. **Presentations and lectures**
   Try to find as many opportunities as you can to speak to people about the services that you offer. This may come in the form of lectures for interested groups or presentations at local health fairs or trade shows. If you are not afraid of public speaking, this can be one of the best ways to allow your audience to get to know you and what you have to offer.

How to price your iridology or nutritional consulting service

The third "P" in your marketing strategy is **PRICE.** Before you begin practicing as an iridologist or nutritional consultant it is important to set the price of your service or products.

1. Your marketing research will assist you in determining what price your clients are willing to pay for your service.
2. Your price should reflect the type of service you are offering, the length of the service as well as your experience in the field.
3. Ask yourself these pricing questions:

a. What will be the cost of a consultation?
b. Will the consultation be based on length of time spent with your client?
c. What will the cost be for a follow-up consultation?
d. Will there be an extra cost for a written iridology or nutritional report?
e. Will you offer discounts to seniors or children?
f. What will be the cost of any nutritional supplements that you offer?

Setting a price is not always the easiest thing to do. For some clients, price will not be an issue at all. For others it will be the major issue when deciding whether to obtain your service. The task that you have is to set a fair price that adequately reflects the service that you will be providing as well as the experience that you have in the field. Remember, you obviously incurred costs for your education, in setting up your practice, in obtaining equipment and other investments, not to mention a lot of investment in time. You need to be adequately rewarded for this. Your price for your service is a reflection of all these investments.

How to find the right place for your iridology or nutritional consulting practice

The fourth and last P in your marketing strategy is **PLACE.** Location is another important factor that you need to address when considering an iridology or nutritional consulting practice.

The beginning iridologist or nutritional consultant often begins their practice from their own home. The advantage is that there are no additional costs to incur; the disadvantage is that you are not in a busy location where clients can easily see you.

When considering a place to locate your practice, consider these factors:

1. Is the location of your practice accessible to your primary market?
2. Is it close to transport, buses, trains, subways or metro stations?
3. Is there adequate parking at or near your practice?
4. Is the cost of rent feasible?
5. Is there room to expand, should your practice grow?
6. Is the location wheelchair accessible?
7. Are the premises quiet?
8. Is there much competition in the same area?

Consider all these factors when choosing a location and carefully assess each one of them. Remember the location you choose may be one that will be with you for many, many years. Choose carefully as changing your location too often can harm your practice and may result in loss of many clients.

Learning from your competition

Your competition is often one of your best sources of marketing information. Take a look at any natural therapy clinics or consulting practices around your area and examine what they are doing and how long they have been in business.

What can you learn from your competition?

You can learn:

- what prices they charge for consultations
- what services they offer

- what type of office they have
- how long they have been in business for
- where they are located

Once you compile this information, you can find ways to possibly improve on your service, make it different and better than the competition. Perhaps you can take a look at their reports that they offer their clients or even make an appointment for yourself to see what they are doing. Information from your competition will also assist you to come up with your own pricing schedule as well as help in finding where you should be located.

It pays to do preliminary research, before you invest in premises, equipment etc. Remember a high percentage of natural therapy clinics do not succeed and this is usually because of poor planning and lack of any marketing research.

How to build a solid client base

The secret to a successful iridology or nutritional consulting practice is to not only attract clients but to keep them coming back and telling their friends. A satisfied customer can be all you need in terms of advertising as word of mouth spreads faster than wildfire. A dissatisfied customer can damage a practice and detract clients from coming. As it is impossible to satisfy everyone, you will always have some clients that are not satisfied with your service. The important thing to remember is that you need to satisfy a high percentage of your primary market.

It is important to maintain a high level of professionalism and high standard of quality in all the consulting work that you do.

Keep these helpful pointers in mind:

1. No one wants to feel like a number but as a person. Treat every client, as you would like to be treated yourself. Give them ample time, empathize with their situation, listen and show compassion.
2. Never put down your competition or say anything negative about them to your clients. It only will show your client that you are not secure with yourself.
3. Using advertising and promotion methods that we have discussed in this module will attract clients and make them aware of your services, but your professional people skills will keep them coming back and recommending you to others.
4. Do not be afraid to recommend your clients see another specialist or doctor if you are not knowledgeable in their condition. Clients will not think anything less of you but will respect you if you are honest with them.
5. Many clients will have questions after their consultation. Allow them to contact you or arrange for a follow-up consultation to monitor their progress. Clients like to feel that you are taking care of them.
6. Ensure that you offer a fair price for your service, that your reports and consulting service you offer are comprehensive and that you satisfies the needs of your clients.

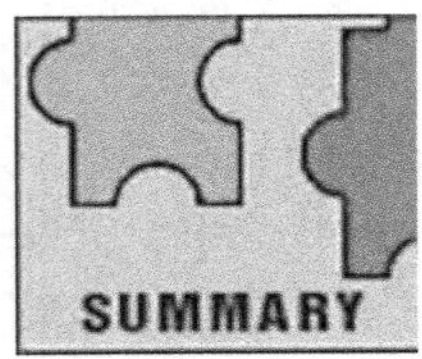

1. Marketing research is simply the study of markets or groups of people that you would like to sell your iridology or nutritional consulting service to. In other words, it is learning about your customers or clients.
2. Your potential clients must all have a particular need, the power to make a decision, finances to obtain your service as well as easy access to your service.
3. When performing marketing research it is important to ask questions, to visualize your ideal client, determine your primary and secondary markets, and to gather information directly from the source.
4. The four P's of any marketing strategy include Product, Promotion, Price and Place.
5. It is important to clarify what your iridology or nutritional consulting service will offer.
6. Methods to promote your practice include various forms of paid and free advertising, trade shows and conferences, as well as presentations and lectures.
7. Your price for your consulting service should reflect the type of service you are offering, the length of the service as well as your experience in the field.
8. Ensure that you carefully choose a location for your practice after considering factors such as costs, parking, transport and competition.

9. Information about your competition is one of the best ways to assist you in making decisions about pricing, type of service and location.
10. The secret to a successful iridology or nutritional consulting practice is to not only attract clients but to keep them coming back and telling their friends. It is important to maintain a high level of professionalism and high standard of quality in all the consulting work that you do as well as utilizing effective people skills.

Please take the time to answer these questions:

1. Explain what is involved in marketing research.
2. List the characteristics of your potential clients
3. List and explain four steps in performing marketing research.
4. What are the 4 P's of marketing? Explain.
5. What are important factors to consider when choosing a location for your practice?
6. List some methods to promote your iridology or nutritional consulting practice.
7. What can you learn from your competition?
8. How can you build a solid client base?

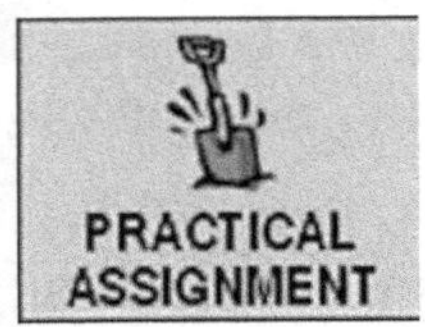

1. Go out and perform the 4 steps of marketing research on your own consulting practice.

   Ask questions as well as put together a survey that you can give to potential clients.
2. Take a close look at the service that you will be offering and write down what it will be comprised of.
3. Research suitable ways that you can advertise your service that will be the most cost-effective.
4. Set and write down all the prices of your services.
5. Analyze the best location for your premises.
6. Do some research about the competition in your geographical area.

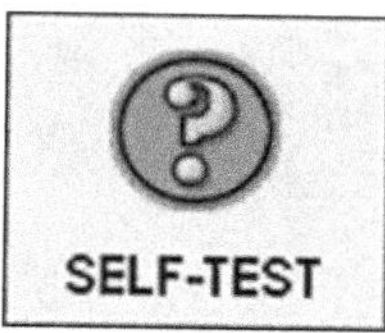

Module 4 Self-Test

1. **Marketing research involves:**
   a) asking questions
   b) visualizing your ideal client
   c) determining your primary and secondary markets
   d) all of the above

2. **Potential clients have all except:**
   a) a particular need
   b) adequate finances
   c) no decision-making authority
   d) easy access to your service

3. **The 4 P's of marketing do not include:**
   a) Price
   b) Precision
   c) Promotion
   d) Place

4. **Relatively inexpensive methods for advertising your service include:**
   a) flyers
   b) free publicity
   c) television
   d) two of the above

5. **Methods of promotion include:**
   a) advertising
   b) trade shows
   c) presentations
   d) all of the above

6. **Factors to consider when choosing a location for your practice include:**
   a) cost of rent
   b) parking and transport
   c) location of competition
   d) all of the above

7. **The first of the 4 P's, Product involves:**
   a) how you will let clients know about your service
   b) clarifying what you will offer to your clients
   c) where you will locate your premises
   d) the costs of your service

8. **The best way to promote your iridology or nutritional consulting practice is by:**
   a) word of mouth
   b) magazine ads
   c) flyers
   d) television advertising

9. **Information about your competition assists in your decisions on:**
   a) price
   b) location of your premises
   c) type of service offered
   d) all of the above

10. **Effective promotion attracts clients to your practice but what best keeps them coming back?**
    a) effective advertising
    b) ads in the local health magazines
    c) professional people skills
    d) low prices

Answers can be found at the end of the book

CHAPTER 5

Developing Your Credibility As A Professional Iridologist Or Nutritional Consultant

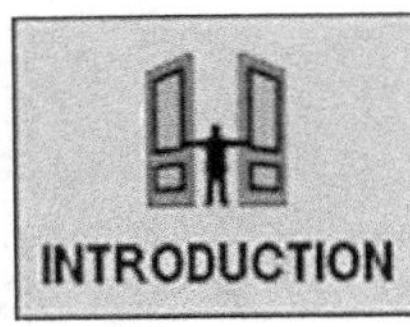

The fifth chapter of this book examines techniques that will develop your credibility as a professional iridologist or nutritional consultant. It includes a discussion of interpersonal skills, professional behavior, confidentiality and lecturing. Included are methods that will build your reputation and professionalism in the field of iridology or nutritional consulting.

At the end of this chapter you should be able to:

- list the factors that are important to develop credibility and professionalism
- appreciate the meaning of professional behavior
- appreciate the value of education

- be familiar with important interpersonal skills
- understand the importance of confidentiality
- appreciate the value of publishing articles and writing
- understand the benefits of effective lecturing and presentations

Before you begin learning methods on how to develop credibility as a professional iridologist or nutritional consultant, it is important to learn what a professional iridologist or nutritional consultant really is.

A professional iridologist or nutritional consultant:

- is one who is sufficiently educated in his or her field as well as related fields
- has sufficient experience dealing with a variety of health problems, their causes, and their treatment and prevention
- has well developed communication skills
- is a good public speaker
- reflects confidence but not arrogance
- is able to positively influence others
- is able to be a leader and role model
- has a passion for his or her profession
- has empathy, respect and compassion for others
- is accepting of others
- is reliable and has the ability to earn trust from clients
- is a teacher and educator
- is one who also practices what he or she preaches

If we want to achieve this level there are certain factors we must adopt to achieve credibility and professionalism:

1. Ensure that your education backs up the level of your service. Ask yourself if you possess any deficiencies and take courses to improve your skills. Never make yourself out to be better than you really are. Being a professional does not mean you have to know everything but to be honest at all times with your clients and with yourself.
2. Gaining experience in the field of iridology and nutritional consulting takes time. It is important that you see a wide range of clients, males, females, young and old with a variety of health problems and conditions. With time, your confidence will grow and you will also find that you will come across similar health problems and your consultation work with clients will give you a rich database of information that you will be able to apply to future situations.
3. As a major portion of your work will be communicating with your clients, this interpersonal skill is something that to some comes naturally, to others it has to be worked on. The better you know how to communicate, the better your relationships with your clients will be. Communication involves active listening to your clients, clearly explaining and educating in order to influence them to make positive diet and lifestyle changes. It is important to talk at the level of your client, not above or below. You will learn to judge what type of client you have and what their level of understanding is so that you can adjust how you will communicate to them. The bottom line is not for you to spill out all you know and show that you are an expert but to transfer your knowledge and experience to others in an effective way that they can understand. It makes no sense for your client to leave confused after a consultation that they hardly understood. Ensure that you

speak clearly and adjust the information according to each individual. Repeat if necessary and ask them if they understand what you are recommending or explaining. In this way you will gain respect and a high degree of credibility.

4. They say that public speaking is one of the most feared activities but it is a skill that you will find is worthwhile to develop. A very effective way to improve your credibility and professionalism in your career is to speak about what you know to others. You may be called on to make a presentation or perform a lecture on iridology or nutrition. This may result in an increase in your client base as well as greater respect in your field. If you are new to public speaking, take a course and start gaining experience. Find local clubs or events like trade shows where you can present your service to groups of people. At one point in time or another, all the great iridologists or natural therapists had to speak to groups of people.
5. A professional reflects confidence but not arrogance. There is a big difference. You can boast about your academic credentials to try to impress your clients but you will not gain their respect that way. A real professional will be confident in their skills but will always listen to others and be willing to learn. Part of the downfall of today's health care system is the arrogance of many medical doctors who do not want to change their attitudes and learn new things. You will not move forward this way. Many patients are afraid to be honest with their doctors because they are just too intimidated by them. Don't fall into this same trap. You have decided to become a professional iridologist or nutritional consultant because you are open to new ideas. Ensure that you stay that way. A closed mind learns nothing new.
6. An important responsibility that you have is that you have the ability to influence others. For this reason, you are responsible for the advice that you offer. A professional has the skill

and experience to positively influence others. In order for your clients to listen and put in practice your advice, they must respect you and what you are saying. They will gain this respect as you build your credibility and professionalism.

7. As a professional iridologist or nutritional consultant, you will be placed in the role of a leader, as you will be an educator with the power to influence and your clients will follow what you say. Again, leadership skills are required such as ability to make concrete decisions, ability to positively influence others and the ability to command respect. These are all characteristics that place you in the leadership role and assist you to gain credibility and professionalism.
8. Nothing is more convincing that someone who is passionate about what they do in their career. The same applies to the career of a professional iridologist and nutritional consultant. If you love what you do and believe in what you are doing, this energy will be felt strongly by your clients and they will be more apt to follow your advice and it will be easier to convince them. Hence you will achieve credibility. I sincerely believe that the power to influence other people's lives is directly related to the level of passion you have in what you are advising.
9. A career in the healing arts should not be about money but about people. These people or your clients are seeking your help and that is why they are there. Having the ability to empathize with their situation and with their problems will earn their trust and belief in your abilities. If you keep in mind that each one of us is different and that these differences should be respected, then you will learn about true human compassion. Being a professional means being compassionate, respecting others and showing empathy.
10. Accepting others is an important characteristic of a professional in the healing arts. We are not any better than anyone

else, we are just different and again these differences need to be respected. For everyone that walks into your office, they have reached this state or situation due to host of reasons and events that are completely different than anyone else. Accept each person as an individual and you will not only achieve success in understanding his or her health problems and causes but you will gain his or her respect.

11. Trust is unfortunately not something that automatically comes with the job of an iridologist or nutritional consultant. Many people are sceptical about iridology or alternative nutritional strategies for prevention and treatment of disease. You need to earn their trust and this depends on a lot of factors. First of all, trust comes with reliability as well as confidence in what you are doing. If you are reliable and confident, if you have the ability to educate and influence others positively and if you respect your clients and utilize effective communication skills, their trust in you will grow. A lack of trust in you and your abilities by your clients often comes with a hidden need to be educated so it is very important that you improve your ability to communicate and teach what you know from your experiences at a level that they can understand.
12. One of the greatest skills of a professional iridologist or nutritional consultant is a strong ability to teach and educate. In order to teach, our clients have to be motivated to listen. A motivating teacher is often hard to find. Work on your teaching skills; ensure that your advice and explanations are clear and easy to understand. Use real-life examples of what you have experienced in the past to make it interesting and motivating for your client. Ensure that the advice you give is achievable and understandable for the client. An excellent teacher is always looked upon as a professional with a high level of credibility.

13. Finally, make sure that you practice what you preach. You have decided to be in the health field and often in the position of making recommendations on diet and lifestyle advice. To gain credibility and respect, you do have an obligation to not only offer quality advice but to practice what you teach your clients. If you are overweight, and advising others of how to lose weight or if you recommend a healthy diet while at the same time you indulge in coffee and donuts all the time, you are not being a good role model. It is very difficult to gain true respect that way.

The importance of confidentiality

An important aspect of professional behavior between a practitioner and a client is confidentiality. As professional iridologists or nutritional consultants you are responsible to maintain confidential what is shared as well as what is learned about the client's health problems. Their iridology report or nutrition report should only be discussed between you and your client. Your client expects the same level of confidentiality as he or she would expect from their medical doctor. Nothing destroys the element of trust in the eyes of a client than failing to maintain confidentiality.

The value of publishing articles

If you have the opportunity to write for a health magazine or publish any articles on the subjects of iridology or nutrition or have special research that you have compiled and wish to share, all this will further your career in your field and will increase your credibility.

The benefits of effective lecturing and presenting

Presentations and lectures on your specialty will increase your reputation as a professional. Utilize every opportunity in your area to speak on your service and you will soon see your practice grow rapidly.

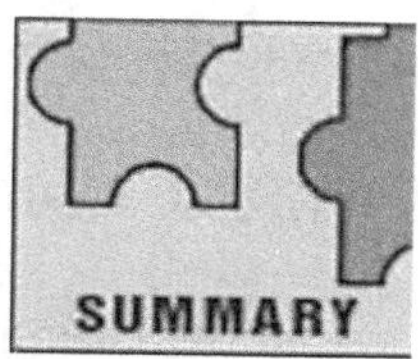

1. A professional iridologist or nutritional consultant is educated and experienced with exceptional communication skills. Confidence, empathy, respect, reliability and leadership are just a few of the many traits that are required to promote credibility and professionalism.
2. Communication involves listening to your clients, clearly explaining, and educating.
3. Ensure that you are assertive and confident in your ability to deal with clients, but avoid arrogant behavior.
4. As a consultant you are in a position of authority and have the ability to strongly influence others. Do not take this responsibility lightly.
5. Utilize your leadership role to positively influence others through your work.
6. Stay true to your beliefs in your profession. Your passion will gain you respect, credibility and a strong following.
7. Respect other human beings and treat them the way that you would like to be treated. Respect individual differences and opinions.

8. Find ways to build trust and win over skeptics. If you are professional and reliable you will soon build trust in your clients.
9. Find creative and interesting methods to communicate with your clients, to hold their attention and to motivate them to make diet and lifestyle changes.
10. Be a role model for your clients. Practice what you preach.
11. Confidentiality is a must in order to build trust and develop a professional environment between you and your client.
12. Publishing articles is a useful method to build credibility in your field.
13. Public speaking in the form of lectures or presentations is another way to build credibility in your profession.

Please take the time to answer these questions:

1. List and explain some traits that make up a professional iridologist or nutritional consultant.
2. Describe the essential components of communication.
3. What is the difference between confidence and arrogance?
4. What power does an iridologist or nutritional consultant have over their clients?
5. What responsibility do they have?
6. How can you win over skeptics and non-believers in your methods?
7. What does it mean to be a role model?
8. What do we mean by confidentiality?
9. What are some techniques that build credibility?

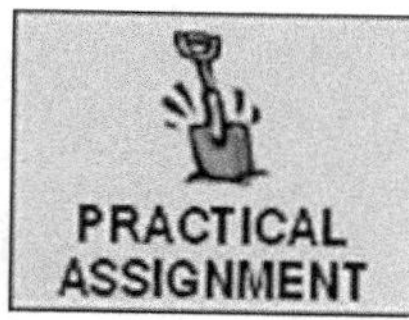

1. Examine the way you communicate to others. Do you listen enough? Practice giving recommendations to clients.
2. Examine your diet and lifestyle habits. In what way can they be improved? Are you practicing what you are preaching? Doing what you preach will make you a better teacher and motivator in your profession.
3. Prepare yourself for skeptics by writing down responses to expected reactions.
4. Write to or call some local health magazines or newspapers and ask them if you can write an article for them.
5. Practice your public speaking skills in front of groups of people.

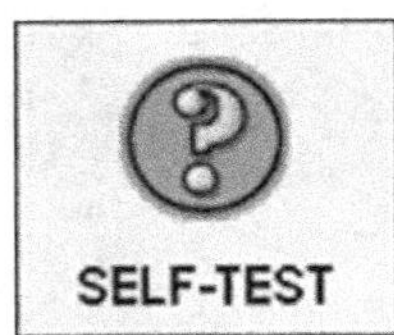

Chapter 5 Self-Test

1. **Effective communication skills include:**
   a) listening
   b) talking above the level of your client
   c) clearly explaining
   d) two of the above

2. **Building trust involves:**
   a) confidentiality
   b) confidence
   c) respect
   d) all of the above

3. **The iridologist or nutritional consultant has a responsibility to:**
   a) utilize arrogant behavior
   b) take advantage of their position of authority
   c) maintain confidentiality
   d) none of the above

4. **Techniques that build credibility include all except:**
   a) presentations
   b) writing articles
   c) practicing what you preach
   d) none of the above

5. **Respecting clients involves:**
   a) accepting who they are
   b) treating them the way you would like to be treated
   c) empathy
   d) all of the above

6. **Motivating your clients to listen your advice includes all except:**
   a) clear explanations
   b) creative teaching skills
   c) lack of passion
   d) experience

7. **A career in the healing arts is most importantly about:**
   a) money
   b) people
   c) advancing your career
   d) building your credibility

8. **In order to gain experience the iridologist or nutritional consultant needs:**
   a) time
   b) to see a wide range of clients
   c) to see a wide range of health problems
   d) all of the above

9. **Your level or degree of service you give should be backed up by:**
   a) the price
   b) your education
   c) your desire to assist
   d) empty promises

10. **To avoid confusion on the part of the client, it is important to:**
    a) Make clear explanations
    b) Listen and ask whether they understand you
    c) Talk at a different level than your client
    d) Two of the above

Answers can be found at the end of the book

CHAPTER 6

Moral, Ethical And Legal Issues That Arise In An Iridology Or Nutritional Consulting Practice

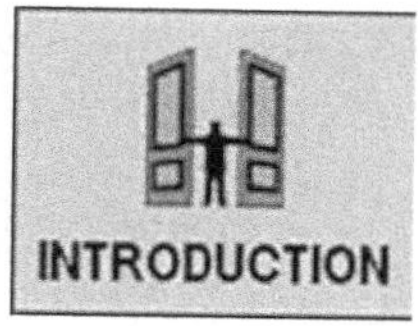

The sixth chapter of this book examines moral, ethical and legal issues related to an iridology or nutritional consulting practice.

At the end of this chapter you should be able to:

- Discuss the essential components of professional ethics
- Be familiar with moral questions that can arise in a clinical setting
- Recognize some of the main moral issues that can confront the practitioner

- Recognize the legal implications for an iridologist or nutritional consultant in diagnosing and treating health problems

Professional ethics

Ethical or moral behavior is an essential component of professionalism in practice. As professional iridologists or nutritional consultants we do not treat diseases or symptoms of a disease, we treat fellow human beings. Each of these human beings is an individual with individual fears, attitudes, opinions, genetic characteristics and ethnic and cultural backgrounds. We as professional iridologists or nutritional consultants need to respect these differences as we are in the healing profession and have a duty to our client.

Good ethical behavior involves following these important guidelines.

1. In trying to do good for others, ensure that you do not harm.
2. As healing professionals, we have a duty to alleviate suffering.
3. Ensure all client iridology or nutritional records are kept confidential and do not disclose any information to a third party without the consent of the client.
4. The interest of the client takes precedence over the interest of the healing professional.
5. Ensure that your education is updated or upgraded and maintained to provide the best possible care for your clients.

6. Ensure that you have consent from your client for any procedure or consultation that you provide.
7. A natural health professional can persuade others to comply with recommendations but should not force a client to comply with them.
8. Do not treat the disease or symptom but treat the whole person.
9. Practice what you preach and be a good role model.
10. We have a duty to promote quality of life that includes mental, spiritual and physical well-being.
11. If the client's needs are beyond your capacity, refer them to a colleague or another specialized professional.
12. If you are not sure of your recommendations, refer your client to someone else for a second opinion.
13. Do not be judgemental. Be loyal to your clients, as this will increase their self-esteem and their confidence in your abilities. Remember, you are there to direct or guide them towards specific health goals and you need their trust and support to accomplish this.
14. Never be under the influence of drugs or alcohol while treating a client and refuse to treat any client who may be under the influence of these substances.
15. Always be truthful to and honest with your clients. Do not promise results.
16. Ensure that your clients are charged fairly for the consultation and that your price reflects accurately your education, training and experience.
17. Never put down or criticize a fellow practitioner or the methods that others use.
18. Never compete for clients by using unethical means to obtain or steal them from other consultants.
19. Do not use misleading advertising to increase your client base.

20. Practice only those modalities in which you are fully trained.
21. Ensure that you are well rested and in good health to ensure the best possible service for your clients.
22. Allow time for relaxation; do not overwork yourself to avoid burnout.
23. Avoid any sexual advances by clients of the opposite sex.
24. Work together as a team with other healing professionals, associations and organizations.
25. Ensure that you are there for the client even after the consultation, if they have any questions or concerns.

Ethical or moral situations that can arise in a clinical setting

Examine the following situations. There are no right or wrong answers to these ethical or moral dilemmas. They are just included here to stimulate thoughts as many are commonly confronted in an iridology or nutritional consulting practice.

1. Your client tells you before their consultation that he or she has cancer and asks how much time does he or she has left to live. What would you say in this situation?
2. After the consultation your client apologizes that he does not have enough money to pay you and goes on to explain all the reasons for his poor state of financial affairs. Will you charge this client?
3. A female client begs you not to tell her husband anything bad about his health status during the consultation or diagnosis because she is afraid that he will not be able to handle it. How would you react?
4. Your client returns several days after his iridology consultation and tells you that you made a big mistake about their health status because their doctor told him that he does not

have any health problems whatsoever and now want his money back from you. How would you react?

5. A young female client tells you during the consultation that her father sexually abused her and that she believes her health problems are a result of this. What would you do?
6. When you complete your iridology analysis, your client asks something about their health for which you do not have an answer. What would you say to them?
7. A client offers to pay you double if you give him better service. Would you take the money? What are possible outcomes if you take the money?
8. A client calls you on the telephone and explains that they have marks on their irises and asks you what they mean. She is very nervous about them as her mother died of cancer. What would you tell her?
9. Your client has only one good eye; the other one is a glass eye. He asks because of this can he have his iris analyzed at half the price. What would you say?
10. A teenager comes for a consultation and asks that you not tell his parents about the results of his examination. His parents call you later and ask about their son's health results. What do you tell them?

Legal implications

As the practice of iridology is not a regulated body in most areas of the world at the time of this writing, it is usually incorporated into certificate or degree programs of naturopathy, natural therapy and alternative medicine or taken alone as a course program. Graduates of these programs or certificates then practice as natural therapists, iridologists, nutritional consultants, naturopaths, natural health consultants or healers. Several iridology associations have been set up but no real international body exists to monitor the practice of iridology to this date. In most areas of the world, iridology is not recognized by conventional medicine and therefore is placed under alternative medicine where legal implications vary from country to country and even state to state. Exceptions are some countries such as Russia where iridology is recognized by the medical profession and even taught at some medical schools.

In some countries you can set yourself up as an iridologist or nutritional consultant without any education or all (obviously not a good idea). Other countries require specific certificates and education as well as insurance in order to open a consulting practice.

For this reason it is important to check with your local authorities on whether you can practice iridology or not and whether you need a special license or specific educational requirements in order to practice. These requirements vary again from country to country.

It is a wise idea if you are able, to obtain personal indemnity and public liability insurance should you ever be confronted with any legal problems.

Some legal issues to consider are:

1. Do not perform any procedure, nutritional consultation or iridology examination without having the consent from your clients. If the clients are under age you should have the consent of their parents. Under no condition should a client be forced against their will in undergoing any consultation or procedure.
2. Just as doctors and medical professionals are required by law to accurately document everything they have done, the

iridology or nutritional consultant should maintain an accurate client record. This includes any nutritional supplements or vitamins that you prescribe, special diets or nutritional assessments and any iridology reports. This not only serves as a legal document but also is very useful for the practitioner to monitor progress and to provide the best service possible.

3. Legal issues are becoming more and more common in medical health care as well as the natural health business so it is recommended to ensure that adequate personal indemnity and public liability insurance cover is obtained for your practice. In some countries it is a requirement in order to join some natural therapy associations.
4. Education and training requirements to be an iridologist or nutritional consultant range from no education in some countries to specific diplomas in others. It is your responsibility to provide the best care for your clients which also means that you should obtain the best training and education possible or what is required for you to practice as an iridology or nutritional consultant in the area that you live. If you confront a legal problem and do not have education to back up what you are doing, you are setting yourself up for trouble.
5. If you are in the practice of prescribing nutritional supplements or vitamins, make sure that you have adequate training for this. Although these items are sold without a prescription, clients can overdose on some and in some clients some supplements or vitamins can evoke negative reactions that the consultant should be familiar with. Ensure that you are trained in recommending nutritional supplements or vitamins and in effects of over dosage.
6. It is a good idea to ensure that your iridology report or nutritional report you give your clients includes a waiver that explains that you are not responsible for any misdiagnosis and that the client should consult with a medical doctor

before engaging in any of the recommended treatments. The reports should state that results and recommendations in the iridology or nutritional report should be used only as a supplement to any conventional diagnosis.

7. Every country has its own requirements to set up a business as an iridologist or nutritional consultant. Often this involves obtaining appropriate business licenses to be able to practice legally. Practicing without a business license when one is required is not recommended as it can lead to possible legal problems.
8. Legal problems often arise due to poor quality of business premises. Ensure that the business location that you operate in is free of any possible dangers or risks to your client. Make sure that the area you work in is safe and is easily accessible for your clients. Ensure that you follow all fire regulations and make sure to maintain hygiene and good air quality. Ensure that any equipment that you use is in good condition and that is does not pose any threat or hazard to your client. This includes iricopes and magnifying lenses, light sources often used in an iridology practice.

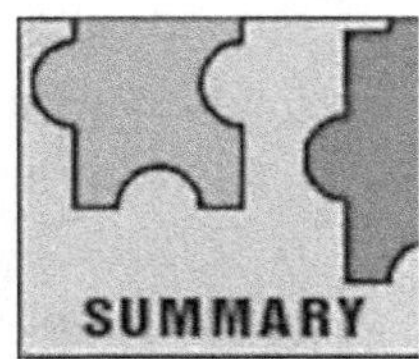

1. Ensure no harm to clients.
2. We have a duty to alleviate suffering.
3. Maintain confidentiality at all times.
4. Place the client's interest as your priority.
5. Update and upgrade your education.
6. Obtain consent from your clients.

7. Persuade clients - do not use force.
8. Treat the whole person.
9. Practice what you preach.
10. Promote quality of life.
11. If not sure refer to a colleague or health professional
12. Do not be judgmental and be loyal to your clients.
13. Avoid drugs or alcohol.
14. Be honest with your clients.
15. Set a fair price for your work.
16. Avoid criticizing other consultants or therapists.
17. Do not obtain clients through unethical means.
18. Do not use misleading advertising to increase your client base.
19. Practice only those modalities in which you are fully trained.
20. Ensure that you are well rested for your work.
21. Take time out to relax to avoid burnout.
22. Avoid sexual advances by clients.
23. Work as a team along with other members of health care.
24. Be there for the client even after their consultation.
25. Ensure that you have informed consent from your clients for any procedure or diagnosis that you perform.
26. Maintain client records, which include their reports, recommended supplements and diets and any advice that you have provided.
27. Ensure, if possible that you are insured in terms of personal indemnity and public liability.
28. Ensure that you have adequate training and education that is required for you to practice in the area that you live.
29. Ensure that you are trained in recommending nutritional supplements or vitamins and in effects of over dosage.
30. Include a waiver in your iridology or nutritional report so that the client is aware of what they are doing and that they are taking any risk onto themselves.

31. Ensure that you have the appropriate business licenses if necessary for your area of the world to practice as an iridologist or nutritional consultant.
32. Ensure that the business location that you operate in is free of any possible dangers or risks to your client in terms of accessibility, fire regulations, hygiene and air quality.

Please take the time to answer these questions:

1. What is meant by professional ethical behavior in an iridology or nutritional consulting practice?
2. List and explain the essential ethical guidelines
3. What should an iridology or nutritional consultant be aware of in terms of legalities?
4. What is required in order to open up an iridology or nutritional consulting practice?

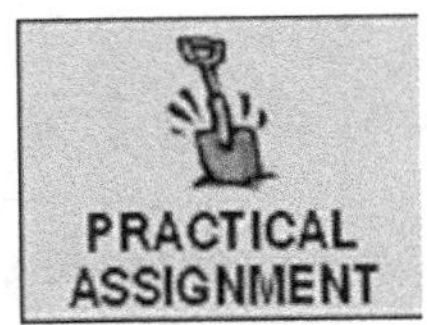

1. Examine each of the guidelines for good ethical behavior and assess whether you are applying them in your work.
2. Develop a system so that you can maintain client records. This may be a file system or even on computer.

3. Research into what business licenses are required in order for you to practice as an iridology or nutritional consultant.
4. Ensure that you obtain the education and training that is required in your country to operate an iridology or nutritional consulting business.

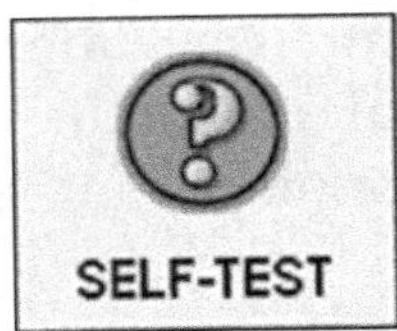

Chapter 6 Self-Test

1. **Good ethical behavior involves all except:**
   a) Maintaining confidentiality
   b) Criticizing other consultants
   c) Setting a fair price
   d) Obtaining consent

2. **An iridologist or nutritional consultant should not be judgmental because:**
   a) each client should be respected
   b) it decreases client's self-esteem
   c) it destroy loyalty
   d) all of the above

3. **A waiver should be included in the consultant's report because:**
   a) it places the responsibility on the client
   b) it places the responsibility on the consultant
   c) it can protect from legal problems should an error occur
   d) two of the above

4. **Business premises should:**
   a) be safe and easily accessible
   b) be clean and hygienic
   c) follow fire regulations
   d) all of the above

5. **An iridology or nutritional consultant should ensure that they:**
   a) possess all required business licenses to perform their work
   b) obtain sufficient education or training
   c) maintain client records
   d) all of the above

6. **Before performing an iridology or nutritional consultation, one should not:**
   a) obtain consent from the client
   b) be under the influence of drugs of alcohol
   c) arrange adequate insurance
   d) ensure safe business premises

7. **Maintaining client records involves all except:**
   a) storing a record of iridology or nutritional reports
   b) storing a record of dietary recommendations or advice given
   c) allowing the client to have the only copy
   d) storing a record of amounts or dosages of supplements prescribed

8. **If you are unsure of your recommendations you should:**
   a) refer your client to a specialist
   b) give what advice you can
   c) pretend that you know what you are doing
   d) all of the above

9. **Ethical guidelines include all except:**
   a) Practice what you preach
   b) Use whatever means you can to obtain clients
   c) Promote quality of life
   d) Treat the whole person

10. **An iridology or nutritional consultant should avoid:**
    a) criticizing other consultants
    b) setting unjustifiable prices for their services
    c) sexual advances by clients of the opposite sex
    d) all of the above

Answers can be found at the end of the book

CHAPTER 7

Professional Iridology And Nutritional Reports

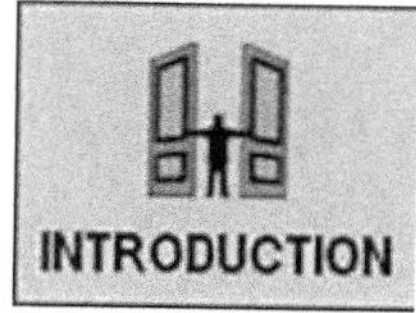

The seventh chapter of this book examines reports related to a professional iridology or nutritional consulting practice.

At the end of this chapter you should be able to:

- Be familiar with the essential components of a professional iridology report
- Be familiar with the essential components of a professional nutritional report

Professional iridology reports

A clear and concise report will develop your reputation as a qualified iridologist. Clients today are increasingly requesting information about their own personal health and providing a high-quality comprehensive report will ensure the utmost professionalism.

Remember a professional iridology report should include the following:

Guidelines in producing a professional Iridology report

1. Include photographs, printed images, or iris drawings with the iridology report. Make sure you keep a copy of the images or photographs for your own records as well as for your client. (Iridology analysis and reporting software is best)
2. If possible label or explain to your clients what iridology signs were found in their eyes.
3. Provide explanations for each of the labeled areas in both irises.
4. Include personal details such as name, telephone, address, age, medications taken, chief complaints, and any eye diseases or operations.
5. Include a short explanation of what iridology is and perhaps something about the history of this branch of alternative medicine. (optional)
6. Provide information on the iris grade of fiber density.

7. Determine the genetic iris constitution and include information in the report on common problems that these eye types experience and what they can expect during their lifetimes.
8. Provide information on how to strengthen the iris constitution depending on what kind of healing methods you provide in your practice.
9. Note colors seen in the iris or sclera and provide possible explanations in your report.
10. Note any iridology signs seen in the pupil, iris, and sclera and provide explanations in your report.
11. Take a look at any lesions in the iris and note the level of tissue change. If you are only using a magnifying glass or photograph, make a judgment based on what you have learned. Note whether the lesion is in an acute, pre-chronic, chronic, degenerative or final stage and provide an explanation for your client. If you are using a computer-assisted program, you will be able to more accurately ascertain changes and to provide a detailed computer report for your clients. The For Your Eyes Only PRO iridology analysis, reporting and scanning software is now available that can scan and record color intensity in areas of the iris, and records this information in graph form, revealing weak body systems and organs etc. Learn more about levels of tissue change in the For Your Eyes Only iridology courses that are available.
12. Take a look at each major body system in the body and summarize the state of health.
13. Never name a disease but provide possible problems that can be encountered by what you see in the human iris. Remember to concentrate on possible causes of health problems rather than outcomes such as symptoms and diseases.

14. Include possible psychological affects that can be encountered or experienced. Remember that every physical deficiency in the body affects the psychological state and vice versa.
15. If you provide healing services such as nutritional therapy, herbal medicine, homeopathy, body therapies or others, note in your report what recommendations you have for the weakened areas that you have seen in the iris.
16. Often many signs will be evident in your analysis, which can result in many existing or potential health problems. You should center on the major health issues in your report so to not confuse the client or scare them with pages of problems. Often it is a good idea to have a section in your report devoted to Primary problems, as well as another section that lists some potential problems to be aware of. In this way the client can concentrate on improving the health status of the major health issues and as is often seen the associated problems often disappear once the major ones are taken care of effectively.

Below is a sample of a professional iridology report. Depending on your needs, this report can be simplified or in even greater detail. You may wish to create your own professional iridology report according to your own requirements. This is only one of many possible formats. To learn more about iridology, genetic constitutions and other information included in this report, take the For Your Eyes Only iridology course and become a Certified Iridologist.

SAMPLE IRIDOLOGY REPORT
Prepared by: Joe Sclera, Iridologist
Prepared for: Client name

Date: January 1, 2004

What is Iridology?

Iridology is a non-invasive method that allows examination of the status of the organs and systems of the body by analysis of the iris, pupil and sclera of the human eye.

About your Iridology Report

Your Iridology report has been prepared to include photos of both your right and left irises and signs that were seen during examination. Included are also summaries of your major body systems and recommendations that can improve your health status.

Client details:

Client Name: Iris Smith
Address: 123 Ciliary St., Pupilville, U.S.A
Telephone: 1234 5678
Age: 40
Eye diseases or operations: none
Medications: antibiotics
Chief complaints: Back pain, frequent bouts of flu, hormonal problems

---

Grade of Iris Fiber Density: Grade D

Explanation: These individuals may have metabolic problems and have difficulty in eliminating waste products from the body. The body is often over-acidic.

Genetic Iris Constitution: Hydro-lymphatic

Explanation:

Physical Iris Description: a blue-to-blue gray iris, which may occasionally be brown with a blurred ring of clouds around the ruff zone as well as another ring of well-defined clouds in the outer ring of the iris. Clouds are often white but may be yellow, orange, or brown depending on degree of toxicity.

General Complaints:

- Chronic lymphatic congestion often with persistent infections
- Commonly suffer from asthma, bronchitis, colds and flu
- There are often weaknesses in the heart with high blood pressure or fluctuations in blood pressure
- Predisposition to rheumatoid arthritis
- Depression, mood changes, and impatience are often seen
- Perspire heavily but suffer from heavy fluid retention which can cause edema and weight fluctuations
- Predisposition to diseases of the urinary tract, urinary infections, gallstone and kidney stone formation and varicose veins
- Often there is minimal endurance

Common Complaints in Childhood:

- Recurrent bronchitis, colds, and flu
- Lymphatic congestion and low immunity to infections
- Prone to allergies

Common Complaints in Adulthood:

- Adults tend to develop a stocky physique with a large abdomen
- Due to fluid problems and edema, they may wake in the morning with a puffy face and eyelids that are swollen
- Cold and damp weather generally worsens their health problems
- Blue-eyed types are more prone to catarrhal problems with heavy mucus secretion like asthma and bronchitis, as well as heart weakness with high blood pressure

Eye colors: White- can indicate inflammation or over-acidity of body tissues

Slight tinge of yellow- can indicate kidney weakness or problems with uric acid metabolism

Pupil Size: Small

Explanation: Parasympathetic nervous system is dominant. There may be slow pulse and greater requirement for quality nutrition. Often goal-oriented, tend to be perfectionists and leaders in society.

Size of Ruff Zone: Relatively small

Explanation: As the pupil is small as well, this indicates you are suited to small meals but energy stores are high as well as endurance. There is lots of drive and ambition, which can stress the adrenal glands and affect circulation.

Pupil flattening: General flattening in the pupils indicating general weakness in the spine with notable Superior lateral flattening in the Left pupil indicating cervical/neck weakness.

Pupil Border: thick, leathery border
Explanation: may indicate stomach problems and poor absorption of nutrients.

Ruff zone/Ruff zone border: jagged, some areas of stricture and ballooned bowel, white border
Explanation: may indicate poor digestion and peristalsis, constipation or diarrhea, inflammation of the autonomic nervous system.

Sclera: no evident signs

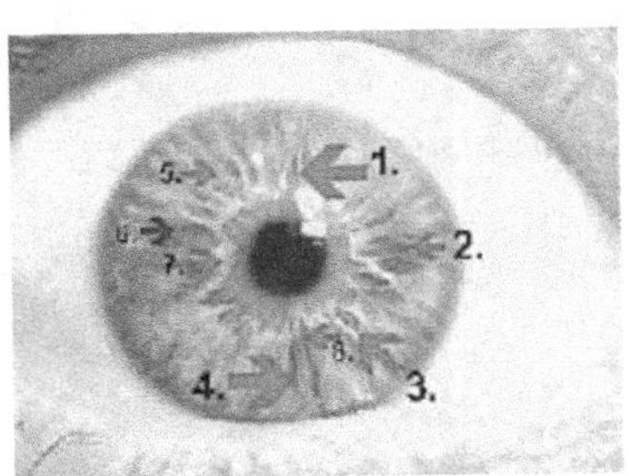

right eye

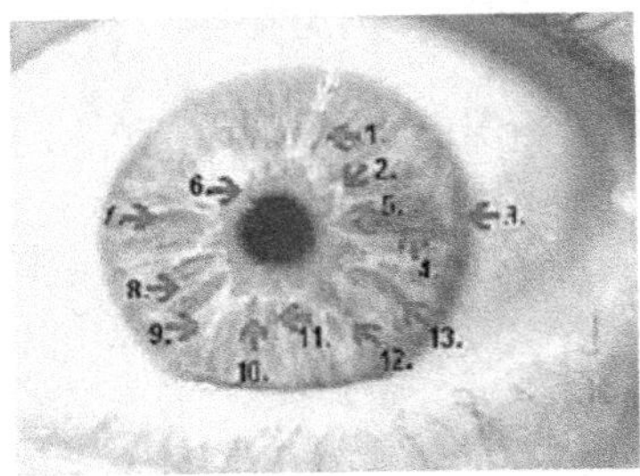

left eye

Iridology signs seen: (numbers correspond to numbered areas in each iris)

Right Eye

1. Weakness in pituitary gland area (pre-chronic)
2. Multiple lacuna indicating chronic weakness in thyroid area, vocal cords and esophagus (chronic/degenerative)

3. Active lacuna in pancreas area (chronic)
4. Right kidney weakness (chronic)
5. Opening of fibers in breathing center and ear zone (acute)
6. Dark area in right lung and bronchial area (pre-chronic)
7. Stricture and distended areas in ascending colon/duodenum
8. Adrenal gland weakness (chronic)

Left Eye

1. Weakness sign in Balance center in brain (pre-chronic)
2. Acute white signs in autonomic nervous system (ruff border)
3. Darkening of ciliary border/ lymphatic clouds
4. Dark area in left lung and bronchial area (pre-chronic)
5. Arc and lacuna in left heart zone
6. White over-acid stomach ring
7. Lacuna in vocal cord/trachea zone (pre-chronic)
8. Sacrum and lumbar spine weakness with activity signs (pre-chronic)
9. White acute inflammation sign in urinary bladder area
10. Weakness sign in uterus area (pre-chronic)
11. Adrenal gland weakness (pre-chronic)
12. Lacuna in spleen area (pre-chronic)
13. Left ovary weakness (pre-chronic)

Summary of state of major body systems:

Glandular: There may be hormonal problems due to weaknesses in the pancreas, thyroid, adrenal, and pituitary glands.

Respiratory: There are weakness signs in both lung and bronchial areas and the breathing center in the brain as well as trachea and vocal cords.

Heart and Circulatory: Weakness signs in the left side of the heart can lead to arrhythmia.

Urogenital: Right kidney weakness, inflammation of the urinary bladder, and weakness in the uterus and left ovary.

Skeletal: Weaknesses in the sacrum, lumbar and cervical spine

Digestive: Over-acid stomach, poor absorption of nutrients, narrowing in ascending colon and ballooned bowel conditions that can lead to poor digestion and constipation/diarrhea

Skin/Lymphatic system: Limited ability of removal of toxins from the skin, acute congested lymphatic system, and weakness in spleen

Sensory organs: Hearing or balance problems may affect right ear

Brain/Nervous system: Breathing center and Balance center may cause problems with breathing or balance. Inflammation/ increased sensitivity of autonomic nervous system can affect digestion.

Summary of six essential processes of life:

Ingestion: quality nutrition is recommended
Digestion: over-acid stomach
Absorption: poor absorption of nutrients
Circulation: left heart weakness
Utilization: weakened hormonal system
Detoxification: kidney, skin and lymphatic system weakness

Summary of Primary problems:

1. Poor absorption and digestion
2. High acidity of body tissues
3. Chronic weakness in the thyroid and pancreas glands
4. Right kidney weakness and inflammation of urinary bladder
5. Respiratory weakness
6. Spinal weakness

Summary of Potential problems:

1. Breathing difficulties/asthma
2. Arthritic conditions
3. Lowered immunity
4. Heart problems
5. Hearing / Balance problems

Conclusions and Recommendations:

It is important that the digestive functions of the body are improved so that the cells receive adequate nutrition. Possible causes of decreased absorptive ability may be high antibiotic use or ingestion of drugs. The high acidity is due in part to genetic constitution but also to weakness of some of the detoxification organs like the kidney, skin and lymphatic system. This may result in problems like fatigue, or joint and spinal problems in older age. Respiratory weakness may be due to smoking or genetic inheritance of weakened lungs or other causes. There are chronic weaknesses in the hormonal glands, which may be caused by stress, poor nutrition, and free radicals generated by the weakened digestive system. The detoxification organs need to be taken care of to improve the level of immunity.

Recommendations:

- Diet? Nutritional Therapy?
- Herbs, vitamins, and minerals?
- Homeopathy?
- Body therapies?
- Other healing methods?

Professional nutritional reports

A clear and concise report will also develop your reputation as a qualified nutritional consultant. Clients today are increasingly requesting information about their own personal health and nutritional advice and providing a high-quality comprehensive report will ensure the utmost professionalism.

Remember a professional nutritional report should include at least some of the following:

Guidelines in producing a professional Nutritional report

1. Include details of the client's nutritional status based on an iridology examination if you are an iridologist or other diagnostic procedure, blood test or direct questions asked. Include personal details such as name, telephone, address, age, medications taken, chief complaints or health problems, and any diseases or operations.
2. If you use iridology in your practice include nutritional advice for genetic iris constitutions (learn more about this in our Holistic Nutrition CD-ROM courses)
3. Include dietary advice and eating plans
4. Include direct nutritional advice for current and potential health problems
5. Include recommendations on nutritional supplements and dosages
6. Include a list of foods to avoid and foods that are beneficial for health
7. Include information on additives to avoid (if applicable)
8. Include specific restrictive diets if required
9. Include cooking advice to maximize nutrients (optional)
10. Include a food pyramid or similar advice to ensure a balanced diet (optional)

Below is a sample of a professional nutritional report. Depending on your needs, this report can be simplified or in even greater detail. You may wish to create your own professional nutritional report according to your own requirements. This is only one of many possible formats. To learn more about holistic nutrition, nutrition for genetic constitutions and other information included in this report, take the Eat Wise by Reading Your Eyes Holistic Nutrition courses and receive your Certificate of Holistic Nutrition.

SAMPLE NUTRITION REPORT
Prepared by: Joe Broccoli, Nutritional Consultant
Prepared for: Client name

Date: January 1, 2004

About your Nutritional Analysis Report

Your Nutritional analysis report has been prepared to include

---

Client details:

Client Name: Janet Vitamin
Address: 123 Apple St., Intestine, U.S.A
Telephone: 1234 5678
Age: 40
operations: none
Medications: antibiotics
Chief complaints: arthritis, heart problems, fatigue

Results from diagnosis

Results from the iridology examination: (if you use iridology, you can include your iridology report)

Blood Test results:

Questionnaire Results: (The answers to specific questions asked can provide a basis for identifying where problems are-)

Genetic Iris Constitution: Hydro-lymphatic type

Nutrition for your Genetic Constitution

Beneficial foods that support your genetic eye constitution

The Hydro-lymphatic constitution is prone to chronic lymphatic congestion and heavy mucus secretion which often lead to low immunity, breathing and heart problems, arthritis and infections.

Again like the Lymphatic Hyper-active constitution it is important to include alkaline foods and to reduce those foods that are mucous forming.

The alkaline-forming minerals include calcium, potassium, sodium, magnesium and iron. Foods that are high in these minerals should be regularly included in the diet. High calcium foods include almonds, egg yolk, green leafy vegetables, soybeans, sesame seeds, parsley and dried figs. High potassium foods include bananas, apricots, avocado, dates, almonds, cashews, pecans, raisins, sardines, and sunflower seeds. High magnesium foods include nuts, whole grain foods, almonds, cashews, molasses, soybeans, spinach, beets, and broccoli. High sodium foods include celery, liver, olives, peas, tuna and sardines. High iron foods include liver, apricots, oysters, parsley, sesame seeds, soybeans, sunflower seeds and almonds.

Excessive lymphatic congestion found in this type necessitates fruits and vegetables that aid in stimulating lymph flow such as apples, watermelon, lemon juice, pineapple, blueberries, grapes, celery, garlic and parsley. Catarrh conditions can be aided with some spices such as cayenne pepper, horseradish and ginger, which boost a sluggish lymphatic system. As the lymphatic system is improved there will be a reduction in rates of infection.

Congestion of the lymphatic system due to improperly digested fats leads to lowered immunity, which means that it is important for the digestion and absorption of fats to work at an optimal rate. This is accomplished by quality bile production from the liver and a healthy intestinal micro floral environment. Liver health can be improved by including foods high in Vitamin C, methionine, choline and inositol. Vitamin C-rich foods include peppers, black currant, broccoli, guava, parsley, pineapple, strawberries, rosehips, raw cabbage, brussel sprouts, and cauliflower. Choline is contained in foods such as beans, egg yolk, lecithin, liver, whole grains and yeast. Inositol containing foods include: beans, corn, nuts, seeds, vegetables, wholegrain cereals and meats. Methionine containing foods include: beans, eggs, garlic, liver, onions, sardines and yogurt. Natural yogurt or soured milk products can restore some of the lost beneficial flora.

As there are often associated heart and circulatory problems such as angina pectoris and high blood pressure, garlic, foods high in calcium and magnesium such as green vegetables, sesame seeds, and almonds should be used frequently in the diet as well as high potassium foods such as bananas, dates, nuts, sunflower seeds, avocado, raisins and apricots. Ensure that you get a good supply of bioflavonoids, which come from cherries, blueberries, black berries and grape juice. This will strengthen veins and capillaries and improve circulation. Include plenty of fiber foods such as vegetables and whole grains to reduce constipation and pressure on veins. Eat plenty of fish especially salmon, tuna and sardines, as they are high in Omega-3 fatty acids, which have been found to be protective of heart function.

Drink plenty of clean water, which is not chlorinated or fluoridated as this can place an extra load of toxins on the kidneys. Cranberries and blueberries are beneficial as they lower calcium levels in urine and may prevent kidney stones. They also help prevent bacteria from adhering to the walls of the urethra and bladder reducing the risk of infection. Eat plenty of watermelon and include lemon juice to prevent kidney stone formation. Include sources of lecithin such as egg yolks, liver, soybean, wheat germ and cabbage as well as olives and olive oil as they help in the digestion of fats and cholesterol and may prevent gallstones.

Beneficial vitamins, minerals, herbs and supplements for your genetic eye constitution

Calcium, potassium, sodium, magnesium and iron are helpful as alkaline-forming minerals. To improve the immune system due to lymphatic congestion, supplements of Vitamin C, E, B-complex, Beta-carotene, Shiitake mushrooms (*Lentinus edodes*), Echinacea, Golden Seal (not during pregnancy) (*Hydrastis canadensis*), Garlic, Bee pollen, Ginseng and Zinc are very beneficial. To improve digestion and absorption of fats and to restore digestive function due to antibiotic use include supplements of Lactobacillus acidophilus, Chlorella and Lecithin. Herbs such as Slippery Elm (*Ulmus fulva*) and liquorice root (*Glycyrrhiza glabra*) are useful in repair of the intestinal mucosa. For joint stiffness and arthritis, it is important to assist liver and digestive function and Glucosamine Sulfate and Chondroitin Sulfate can be beneficial in improving the lubrication of joints and regeneration of joint tissue. Evening primrose oil, and Omega-3 fish oils also assist arthritic conditions. For high blood pressure and heart conditions, Omega-3 fatty acids, coenzyme Q-10, lysine and Vitamin C, E and bioflavonoids such as rutin or hesperidin are very beneficial. Herbs such as garlic, gingko biloba, ginseng and hawthorn berry (*Crataegus monogyna*) have been known to stabilize blood pressure and improve circulation.

Other important advice for your genetic eye constitution

Milk products should also be avoided as there are commonly allergies to milk lactose and they can cause an overproduction of mucous which can produce allergies or respiratory problems especially in the nose, throat, ear and lung areas. Other mucous-forming foods that should be avoided are refined grains such as white bread, cakes as well as white sugar. The intake of caffeine, sugar, salt, dairy foods and alcohol also contribute to lymphatic stagnation.

As there are often very congested lymphatic glands, regular exercise is particularly recommended for better lymphatic circulation. Swimming is particularly helpful for asthmatic conditions or breathing difficulties. Regular lymphatic massage is recommended to stimulate lymphatic flow.

Avoid too many acid-forming foods such as excess meats, saturated fats and citrus fruits that are picked before they are ripe. This will improve arthritic conditions.

Avoid cough suppressants as coughing helps get rid of mucous. Practice deep-breathing exercises and avoid smoking and smoky or smoggy environments if you suffer from respiratory conditions such as bronchitis or asthma.

Maintain adequate water intake and reduce salt, especially hidden salt found in many processed foods in order to prevent fluid retention in the body.

Nutrition to address chief complaints

For arthritis:

Ensure beneficial foods for arthritis such as alkaline foods that include plenty of vegetables, seaweed, parsley, carrots, almonds, blackberries, olive oil, sesame seeds, celery, bananas, avocado, alfalfa sprouts, kelp, brown rice, seeds, garlic, onions, figs and cherries.

Eat plenty of salmon, tuna, mackerel and sardines, as they are rich sources of beneficial fats that decrease inflammation and tissue destruction.

Include foods high in antioxidants, especially those high in beta-carotene, Vitamin C and E. and in the liver and kidney nutrients, methionine, choline and inositol.

Drink celery and carrot juice.

Avoid acid-producing foods such as sugar, white flour, meat, refined carbohydrates and saturated fats.

Avoid milk products other than soured milk or natural yogurt.

Reduce meat intake as meat has a high phosphorus-to-calcium ratio that can have negative effects on the body if taken in excess and it increases acidity.

Avoid salt, coffee, alcohol, vinegar and citrus fruits (except lemons)

Be careful of artificial flavors, colors and preservatives in the foods that you eat.

Drink plenty of "live" water free of chlorine and fluoride.

Avoid using aspirin or other anti-inflammatory drugs.

Supplements such as Lactobacillus acidophilus, Chlorela and Slippery Elm bark (*Ulmus fulva*) assist the Leaky gut syndrome and reduce free radical formation, lecithin and milk thistle (*Silybum marianum*) for the kidney and liver, and Cod liver supplements, Yucca, B-complex, Omega-3 fatty acids, Vitamin C, E, Glucosamine sulfate, chondroitin sulfate and Evening Primrose oil have all been found to benefit regeneration of tissue and reduce inflammation in the arthritic patient. **Recommended dosages for nutritional supplements: ????**

Some anti-inflammatory herbs that can assist with inflammation and pain are Angelica (*Angelica archangelica*), Black Cohosh (*Cimicifuga racemosa*), Feverfew (*Chrysanthemum parthenium*), Ginger (*Zingiber officinale*), Bromelain, a chemical in pineapple and Wild Yam (*Dioscorea villosa*)

Engage in regular exercise preferably swimming as it places the least strain on the joints.

For heart problems:

Increase your intake of fish especially salmon, tuna and sardines, as they are high in Omega-3 fatty acids that reduce the risk of heart disease.

Increase your intake of fruits and vegetables especially those high in Vitamin C and beta-carotene.

Reduce the amount of saturated fat, which means reducing animal fats from meat, cheese and milk products. Saturated fats increase platelet aggregation (binding together) as well as increasing the chance of embolism, while polyunsaturated fats, particularly lineolic and linolenic acids, have the opposite effect.

Strengthen the liver to assist bile production so that cholesterol metabolism in the body is improved. Include foods high in methionine, choline, inositol and Vitamin C and use olive oil regularly. Include herbs such as Milk thistle (*Silybum marianum*) and dandelion (*Taraxacum officinale*) to improve liver function.

Other supplements that can assist in heart disease are: Garlic, Omega-3 fatty acids, Vitamin C, Natural Vitamin E, lysine, chromium, magnesium, potassium, gingko biloba, psyllium, soy lecithin, Co-enzyme Q-10 and Vitamin B-complex. **Recommended dosages for nutritional supplements: ????**

Eliminate sugar and refined flour from the diet and avoid preservatives, colors and artificial flavors in foods.

Avoid trans fatty acids that are found in hydrogenated vegetable oils such as margarines and vegetable shortenings. Avoid fried foods.

Ensure complex carbohydrates and adequate fiber in the diet.

Drink plenty of "live" water free of chlorine and fluoride and avoid coffee.

Include garlic, onions, ginger and alfalfa regularly in the diet as they can inhibit clot formation and reduce cholesterol deposits.

Engage in regular exercise to strengthen the cardiovascular system and to prevent obesity.

Avoid smoking and excess alcohol, which have been found to be significant risk factors for heart disease.

Avoid excess salt and watch out for hidden salt found in most processed foods.

Use relaxation methods to deal with the build-up of stress, which can have negative effects on the heart.

For fatigue:

Ensure that you support all the detoxification organs of the body. Include foods high in methionine, choline and inositol and Vitamin C for the liver and the kidneys and assist bowel function with natural yogurt or soured milk products.

Supplements that will assist in detoxification of the body include Lactobacillus acidophilus, Chlorella and Slippery Elm bark (*Ulmus fulva*) to aid in digestion and absorption as well as lecithin for the liver, kidneys and nervous system. The antioxidant vitamins C, E, beta-carotene and selenium can counteract free radical formation.

Assist the immune system and liver function by including supplements of Echinacea, dandelion (*Taraxacum officinale*), milk thistle (*Silybum marianum*) Golden Seal (not during pregnancy), Shiitake (*Lentinus edodes*) and Maitake mushrooms (*Grifola frondosa*) and Garlic.

Herbs such as Gingko biloba are beneficial for circulation especially to the brain area and bioflavonoids (rutin or hesperidin) found in skins of fruits and vegetables and berries or as supplements will assist in strengthening the capillaries.

To improve energy levels ensure foods high in Vitamin B-complex, Vitamin C, Iron, magnesium and beta-carotene. Supplements of Coenzyme Q-10 can also assist. **Recommended dosages for nutritional supplements: ????**

Eat smaller meals five times a day.

Ensure adequate rest and moderate exercise, but not to the point of exhaustion.

Perform five minutes of deep breathing exercises every day.

Reduce stress in your daily life and do not push yourself too hard.

Do not smoke.

Have your amalgam fillings removed by a specialist who knows what they are doing.

Suggested sample eating plan

Before breakfast – large glass of water with fresh lemon juice

Breakfast – Fresh fruit salad (include apples, watermelon, pineapple, grapes, bananas, blackberries) with natural yogurt

Before Morning Snack – large glass of water

Morning Snack – raisins, sunflower seeds, almonds

Before lunch –large glass of water

Lunch – sardines, wholegrain roll, fresh raw salad (include parsley, celery, sesame seeds, fresh peas, olives, spinach, beets, peppers, corn, onions, garlic, olive oil, cayenne pepper)

Before afternoon snack – large glass of water / grape juice

Afternoon snack – dried figs, apricots, celery

Before Dinner – large glass of water / fresh apple and celery juice

Dinner – Slice of turkey with cranberries and brussel sprouts or broccoli, raw salad (include cabbage, peppers, parsley, avocado, celery, cucumber), cherries for dessert

Before After Dinner Snack – large glass of water

After Dinner Snack – dates, grapes

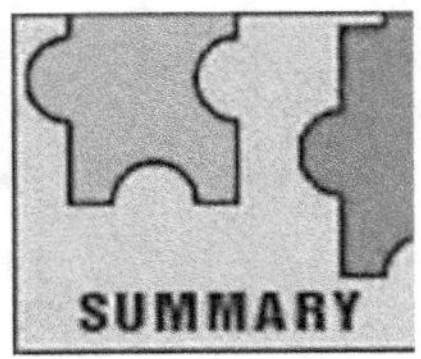

A professional iridology report should include:

- photographs, printed images, or iris drawings
- an explanation of iridology signs found in the eyes
- personal details, medications taken, chief complaints, and any diseases or operations
- a short explanation of what iridology is
- information on the iris grade of fiber density
- the genetic iris constitution and common problems
- information on how to strengthen the iris constitution
- colors seen in the iris or sclera
- iridology signs seen in the pupil, iris, and sclera
- lesions in the iris level of tissue change.
- a summary of each major body system in the body
- include possible causes of health problems, not symptoms and diseases
- possible psychological states
- recommendations for weakened areas that you see in the iris
- include sections for primary problems and potential problems

A professional nutritional report should include:

- details of the client's nutritional status
- personal details, medications taken, chief complaints, diseases or operations
- nutritional advice for genetic iris constitutions
- dietary advice and eating plans
- nutritional advice for current and potential health problems
- recommendations on nutritional supplements and dosages
- foods to avoid and foods that are beneficial
- additives to avoid
- specific restrictive diets
- cooking advice
- food pyramids or advice to ensure a balanced diet

Please take the time to answer these questions:

1. Why is it important in your iridology report to include a photograph or printed image of your client's eyes?
2. List the important components that comprise a professional iridology report.
3. List the important components that comprise a professional nutritional report.

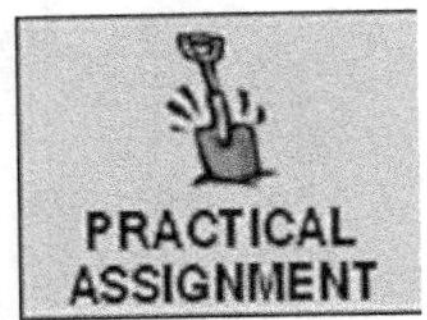

1. Make an outline for an iridology report that you would like to use.
2. Design your own nutritional report.
3. Write down a list of questions that you would ask your client in order to gain more insight into their nutritional status.

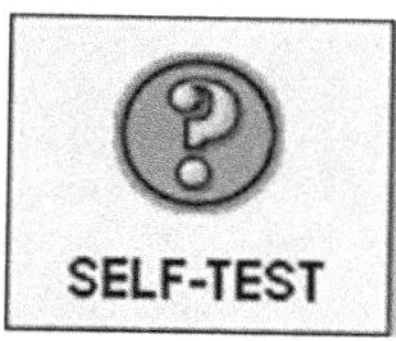

Chapter 7 Self-Test

1. **An iridology report should include all except:**
   a) Explanations of iridology signs
   b) Client details
   c) Diseases
   d) Summary of body systems

2. **Nutritional needs can be ascertained by:**
   a) An iridology examination
   b) Blood tests
   c) Direct questions
   d) All of the above

3. **The iridology report should center on:**
   a) Primary health problems
   b) Potential health problems
   c) Every minor detail of health problems
   d) Two of the above

4. **Nutritional recommendations should be given for:**
   a) Chief complaints
   b) Primary health problems
   c) Potential health problems
   d) All of the above

5. **The iridology report should explain:**
   a) Diseases found
   b) Causes of diseases
   c) Symptoms found
   d) None of the above

6. **An ideal nutritional report will provide nutritional advice for:**
   a) Genetic constitution
   b) Chief complaints
   c) Potential health problems
   d) All of the above

7. **In addition to nutritional recommendations it is wise to include:**
   a) Food additives to avoid
   b) Eating plans
   c) Beneficial foods
   d) All of the above

8. **A clear and concise report is important because of all except:**
   a) It is professional
   b) It ensures that clients will adhere to your advice
   c) It is faster to produce
   d) Clients demand information and advice that is easily and clearly understood

9. **Which of the following is not a component of a professional iridology report?**
   a) Explanation of colors and signs seen in the iris, pupil and sclera
   b) Description of the genetic iris constitution
   c) Information on the grade of iris fiber density
   d) Inclusion of diseases that exist or could potentially occur

10. **Which of the following is not a component of a professional nutritional report?**
    a) Nutritional advice for primary health problems
    b) Eating plans
    c) Miracle overnight weight loss programs
    d) Nutritional status

Answers can be found at the end of the book

CHAPTER 8

The Iridology Or Nutritional Consultation

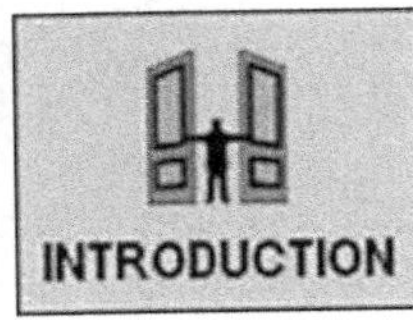

The eighth chapter of this book examines what is involved in an iridology or nutritional consultation, as well as the client-consultant relationship.

At the end of this chapter you should be able to:

- Appreciate what clients expect from an iridology or nutritional consultation
- Understand some important components in developing a client-consultant relationship
- Be familiar with ways in which to reduce fear or anxiety during the consultation
- Appreciate the need for confidentiality
- See the importance of developing active listening skills
- Understand the need and role of feedback and follow-up

The iridology or nutritional consultation

What really happens during an iridology or nutritional consultation? What do clients expect from the consultation?

In my many years of experience in consulting with thousands of patients, I have learned a great deal in terms of what clients require, need or expect from iridology or nutritional consulting services. Many have come who have been disappointed with previous consultations with other iridologists or nutritional consultants. If you approach the consultation in a professional manner as described in this course, you will achieve successful results and your clients will keep coming back and refer you to others.

First of all, your clients require information, not too much so that their heads becomes too full and overloaded and not too little that they still have a list of questions at the end of the consultation. Each individual client is different. Some are satisfied with just what they should do to get healthy. Others want to know all the details. You will, with experience learn to assess what type of client you have and adjust to their requirements. The information you give them has to be understandable. You cannot ramble on about anatomy and physiology to someone who does not have a clue about it. The information you give should be concise and clear to the point. Make sure that you ask them if they understand several times to make sure that you can continue. Repeat your recommendations, and summarize them at the end of your consultation so that they know what health problems they have and what they need to work on to get better.

Part of your iridology consultation will be gathering information by either using a magnifying lens to examine the iris or if you have a digital iriscope camera you will be photographing the irises, scanning or analyzing them using iridology software and developing professional reports. With practice and time, an iridology report can be generated in 15 minutes and a multi-page complete analysis can be printed out for the client. Refer back to Module 3 if you are interested to learn more about iridology equipment and software. The standard sequence of events when a client of mine arrives for a personal consultation is that I first of all photograph both irises and save them in a file. They return to the waiting room while I analyze the irises and produce a report. After 15 minutes or so the patient is called in and the rest of the consultation time is used to explain findings and to make recommendations. I ensure that I use the computer screen to show the client the images of their irises and identify what and where the problem areas are. Another option is to photograph the irises one day and ask the clients to return after you have their reports completed. Although not as desirable for most patients, this does allow you in the initial stages to have more time to prepare your report and what you will say in your consultation.

For nutritional consultations, they can be combined with the iridology examination. If you do not use iridology as a diagnostic tool, your nutritional consultation is often spent asking specific questions and listening to the client's problems. After a thorough investigation is made of their health and nutritional status, you can then offer nutritional advice, set them up on special diets, recommend nutritional supplements and other lifestyle advice. If you have nutritional software, you will be able to produce a report for your client, complete with nutritional recommendations.

Giving your clients a report so that they can read about it later is a great advantage. Most clients will forget at least 50 percent of what you tell them in the consultation. Having their report in hand will allow them to browse through it in their own time and at their own pace. It will allow them to digest what you have discovered and what you have explained to them. Patient compliance to your health recommendations is greatly increased if they are provided with a clear and concise report

How long should the consultation last?

It is common for a consultation to be between a half an hour to an hour. Anything longer than that, and you will risk that your patient will complain of information overload. Remember, be concise and to the point.

Address their chief complaints

Do not overlook their chief complaints. You may find other health problems in your iridology or nutritional assessment but make sure that you address their primary complaints. This is something that they will demand. Ensure that your recommendations include what they have to do so that these health problems that they are complaining about can improve. If the cause of their health problems is somewhere else, make sure that you explain how it relates to their chief complaints. Again, always repeat and ask your clients if they understand and if you have answered their questions adequately.

The client-consultant relationship

Developing a client-consultant relationship is of the utmost importance when one is practicing iridology or nutrition. A positive relationship can result in greater adherence to treatment or recommendations that you prescribe. It will also allow your client to be truthful about their health problems and open to making changes. Let's face it, in this business; one of the hardest things for clients to do is to follow your guidelines and recommendations and to make a change for the better. The way you approach and relate to your client will often determine whether the client is successful and actually returns to better health or whether they allow their chronic health problems to persist. A negative relationship may result in your clients doing the opposite of what you tell them.

How can we build a positive client-consultant relationship?

Gain mutual respect

Well, first of all we need to gain respect from our client. To do this we have to be professional, we have to believe in what we are doing and recommending. Patients are very sensitive to this and if they feel that you do not really believe in what you are saying, they will not comply with the treatment. If we give our client the respect and care that they deserve, they will reciprocate and give you the respect you deserve. This mutual understanding of each other's needs and each other's role will start to build trust. Once your client has trust in your abilities, they will open up and make it a lot easier for you to make recommendations and to see positive results in their health status.

Be assertive and confident

Our ultimate goal is to have our clients understand what we advise them and to comply with the recommendations that we give them. In order for them to do this they need to feel confident in your abilities. If you come across as someone who is unsure or confused, this will not foster a positive environment. Ensure that you always emit a sense of healthy assertiveness and confidence (without appearing arrogant or insensitive) and your client will feel this radiate from you and will be much more inspired and motivated to make changes in their diet and lifestyle. Clients need to feel the conviction in your voice and the belief in what you are saying to them.

Show empathy not sympathy

When we show sympathy, we feel sorry for another. When we show empathy, we actually share the experience of another. Our clients need to feel understood and by showing empathy, we communicate to them that we care about them and share their feelings, but we do not feel sorry for them. This is a very positive situation and opens the way to build trust and compliance.

How to reduce fear or anxiety

Many clients are very apprehensive about going for an iridology or nutritional consultation. For many, it will be the first time that they have attempted this kind of diagnosis and they don't know what to expect. Often they are afraid that you will uncover something bad so it is important to reassure them that knowledge about their health status will give them the power to overcome their health problems. Make sure that you explain the entire procedure to them and what will go on in the consultation. This will usually place them at ease once they are informed and they will be much more able to communicate freely with you.

Never mention any words such as terminal diseases or cancer as these can instill great fear in people and as an iridologist you are there to find causes of disease, not diseases themselves.

Explain to them that you are there to assist them, to inform them of any health problems and to provide a plan or program that will get them back on the road to health. The client and consultant are a team that works together so that positive things begin to happen. It is your responsibility to create an environment for your client that is free of fear or anxiety.

Maintaining confidentiality

What is shared between the client and the consultant should be kept confidential. If you maintain confidentiality, your clients will trust you, believe in you and listen and comply with your health recommendations. This atmosphere will allow them to feel at ease with you and allow them to open up and share all their problems.

Keeping this in mind, never send your clients their iridology or nutritional report via someone else without their permission. I have even experienced married couples who wish to have separate consultations and keep their results confidential, so make sure you always respect this.

Listening skills

Listening is probably the most important factor when it comes to client-consultant relationships. Often this is a skill forgotten by many modern health professionals. Being able to listen is a valuable tool that will assist you in making valid recommendations for your client.

Ensure that you maintain good eye contact while listening to your client. It is often not easy to actively listen and we have a tendency to always do the talking. Avoid any distractions such as telephone calls while listening to your client. By listening we will show our empathy and this will build trust so that our clients can be open with us and honest.

Some remarkable things begin to happen once your client feels that you are listening to them. Any kind of tension they may have been feeling such as frustration or confusion is released, and they begin to feel that they are not alone in all this and that there is hope.

A good listener is one who is patient, caring, understanding, sensitive and tolerant of others. Make sure that you place listening skills on the top of your list of building a positive client-consultant relationship.

Feedback and follow-up

As mentioned earlier, it is important to know whether your client understands what you are saying. Often they will not say anything, which is a good indication that they are confused or overloaded with information. Several times, during the consultation it is a good idea to ask your client if they understand everything you have said so far or even better to summarize your findings and recommendations. Getting feedback from your clients will let you know where you are at and this is crucial in achieving your ultimate goal: compliance.

In a lot of cases the client may not have any questions during the consultation but they may come later after they go home and read over their reports. Ensure that you offer them the opportunity of follow-up support so that they can call and ask questions.

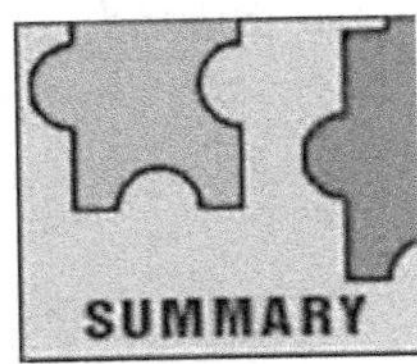

1. Your clients require clear and concise information, not too much so that their heads become too full and overloaded and not too little that they still have a list of questions at the end of the consultation.
2. Giving your clients a report so that they can read about it later is a great advantage and improves compliance.
3. Ensure that the consultation is not too long. Usually a maximum of one hour is sufficient.
4. Your clients will demand that you address their chief complaints.
5. Building a positive client-consultant relationship involves gaining mutual respect, being assertive and confidant and showing empathy.
6. Informing the client what is expected of them during the procedure can relieve fear and anxiety.
7. What is shared between the client and the consultant should be kept confidential.
8. A good listener is one who is patient, caring, understanding, sensitive and tolerant of others. Make sure that you place listening skills on the top of your list of building a positive client-consultant relationship.

9. Ensure that you offer your clients the opportunity of follow-up support so that they can call and ask questions and clear up any misunderstandings.

Please take the time to answer these questions:

1. What comprises an iridology or nutritional consultation?
2. What are some important factors in building a positive client-consultant relationship?
3. What methods would you use to reduce fear or anxiety?
4. Why are listening skills so important during an iridology or nutritional consultation?
5. What is meant by feedback or follow-up?

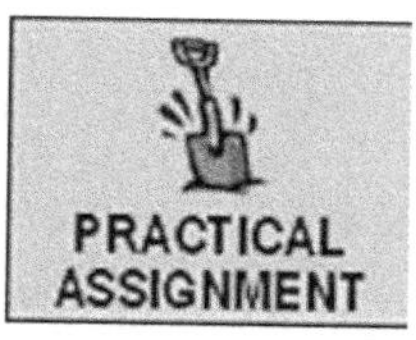

1. Make a plan of what you will actually do in your iridology or nutritional consultation.
2. Practice actively listening to someone and note the results.
3. Practice making a clear and concise presentation or explanation of what you will say in your consultation.

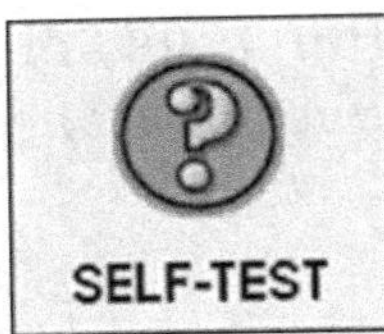

Chapter 8 Self-Test

1. **An iridology or nutritional report:**
   a) is not very useful
   b) is beneficial
   c) improves patient compliance
   d) two of the above

2. **The ideal length of time spent during an iridology or nutritional consultation should be:**
   a) 15 minutes
   b) 2 hours
   c) a maximum of 1 hour
   d) 3 hours

3. **Clients often demand that you:**
   a) not be honest with them
   b) address their chief complaints
   c) give them a reduction in price
   d) none of the above

4. **Building a positive client-consultant relationship involves:**
   a) gaining mutual respect
   b) being confident and assertive
   c) showing empathy
   d) all of the above

5. **Fear and anxiety in the client is often a result of:**
   a) fear of finding out something bad
   b) having too much information
   c) not having enough information
   d) two of the above

6. **Confidentiality is important because it:**
   a) instills trust
   b) improves compliance
   c) places the client at ease
   d) all of the above

7. **Attributes of a good listener include being:**
   a) misunderstanding
   b) patient
   c) insensitive
   d) intolerant

8. **Receiving feedback is essential during your consultation because of all <u>except</u>:**
   a) it ensures that clients understand what you are saying
   b) it improves compliance
   c) it reduces compliance
   d) it allows you to understand the needs of the client

9. **Follow-up is important because?**
   a) it gives clients the opportunity to ask questions at a later time
   b) it stops questions being asked at a later time
   c) it reduces the effectiveness of the client-consultant relationship
   d) None of the above

10. **Each and every client:**
    a) is an individual with individual needs
    b) needs information and advice
    c) should receive respect
    d) All of the above

Answers can be found at the end of the book

CHAPTER 9

Continuing Education For The Iridologist Or Nutritional Consultant

The ninth chapter of this book examines educational requirements and recommended continuing education for the professional iridologist and nutritional consultant.

At the end of this chapter you should be able to:

- Understand the recommended educational requirements to be an iridologist or nutritional consultant
- Appreciate the value of continuing education
- Be familiar with a variety of iridology and nutrition educational resources

Recommended educational requirements for the iridology or nutritional consultant

What does it take to be a professional iridologist?

STEP 1: Get some basic anatomy and physiology education (optional but recommended)

First of all, you will need some education and training in the field. Prior to taking an iridology course or nutrition course, I recommend that you get some basic anatomy and physiology education if you don't already have it. If you are going to talk about the body and health you need to first know something about how it works. This will later be invaluable when you study iridology or nutrition as so much is about body systems and organs and a basic understanding of anatomy and physiology will serve to enhance your understanding of iridology and of human nutritional needs.

There are many anatomy and physiology courses out there and it really does not matter which one you take as long as it covers all the body systems including the:

- Respiratory system
- Heart and circulatory system
- Brain and nervous system
- Digestive system
- Hormonal system
- Skin, tissues and organs

- Detoxification organs
- Lymphatic system
- Renal system
- Liver, gallbladder and pancreas
- Muscular system
- Skeletal system
- Reproductive system
- Immune system
- Human sensory system- sight, touch, smell, taste and hearing

It is also recommended that you have some understanding of concepts such as:

- blood pressure
- the human nerve impulse
- body temperature and metabolism
- muscular contraction
- ageing
- the human cell

STEP 2: Take an iridology / human nutrition course

There are many iridology courses and nutrition courses available, some that teach specific methods, some are home-study courses and others are regular classes. Whichever you choose ensure that the courses cover a good range of material presented in a straightforward and clear manner. Ensure that you check with your local area as to what educational requirements are necessary for you to practice as an iridologist or nutritional consultant. There are many types of iridology methods most popular being the American method, European method or combinations of both American and European.

If you are looking for a good efficient way to learn and take a comprehensive iridology or nutrition home-study course, we recommend the **For Your Eyes Only Iridology courses** or the **Eat Wise by Reading Your Eyes Holistic Nutrition courses.** These three level courses allow you to start from no knowledge of iridology or nutrition and progress through reading assignments, examining iris images, practical and written assignments and self-tests, to a level where you can achieve your **"Certified Iridologist"** certificate or **"Certificate of Holistic Nutrition."**

STEP 3: Get some practical experience

This is not as easy as it sounds but probably the greatest amount of learning that you will get is through practical experience.

A couple suggestions that I would recommend in order to get some practical experience:

- Find an iridologist and ask if you can observe their work and sit in on some of their iridology examinations (often not that easy)
- Start with examining close friends and relatives and practice performing a consultation with them (much more easier)

Continuing education

Education for the professional iridologist or nutritional consultant should never stop. Part of your job should be to continue learning more and more about your field or branch out into other fields of natural medicine.

Sources of information include:

- The Internet- there is ample information about iridology and nutrition there
- Newspapers
- Books

Recommended books on iridology include those written by Josef Deck, Josef Angerer, Bernard Jensen, Theodor Kriege and other world-renowned iridologists

Please read my books, **Iridology: For Your Eyes Only** and **Eat Wise by Reading Your Eyes**

- Magazines on health or alternative medicine
- Journals and research articles

  Journal of Nutritional Medicine, JAMA, Medline, International Clinical Nutrition Review and others
- Additional courses in iridology or nutrition
- Courses in symptomology, disease, holistic medicine and other forms of diagnosis

Other Iridology or Nutrition Education Resources

I have written and developed a broad range of iridology and nutrition education resources for the professional and advanced students of iridology and nutrition.

These include:

1. 100 Iris Case Studies

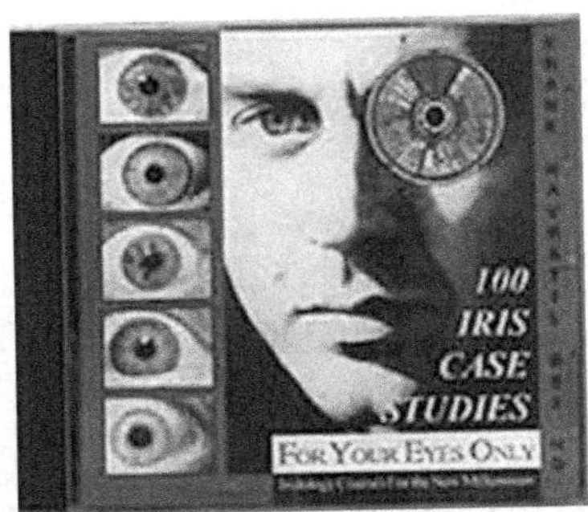

FOR YOUR EYES ONLY - 100 CASE STUDIES
www.irisdiagnosis.org

2. Genetic Eye Constitutions

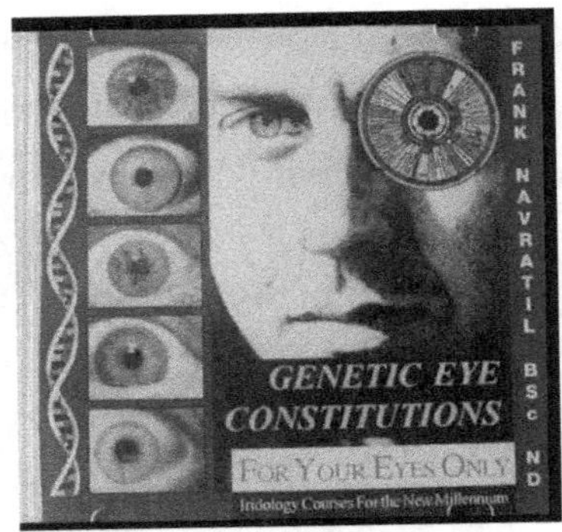

FOR YOUR EYES ONLY -
GENETIC EYE CONSTITUTIONS
www.irisdiagnosis.org

3. Iris, Pupil, Sclera Signs

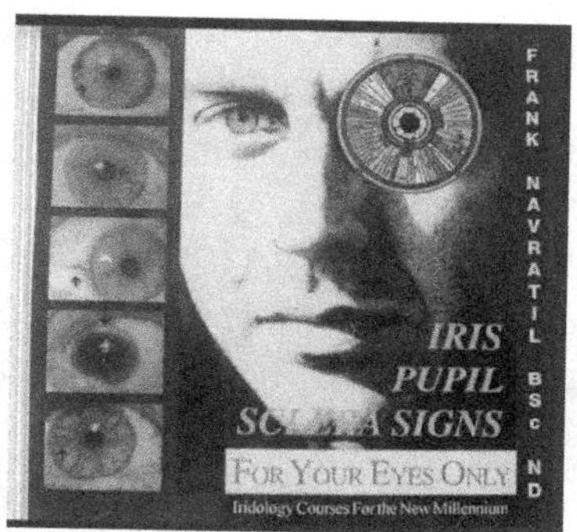

FOR YOUR EYES ONLY -
IRIS, PUPIL AND SCLERA SIGNS
www.irisdiagnosis.org

4. The Brown-Eye Iridologist

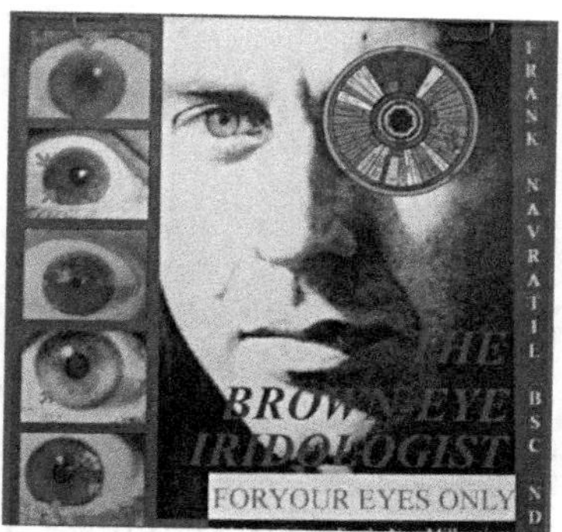

FOR YOUR EYES ONLY -
THE BROWN-EYE IRIDOLOGIST
www.irisdiagnosis.org

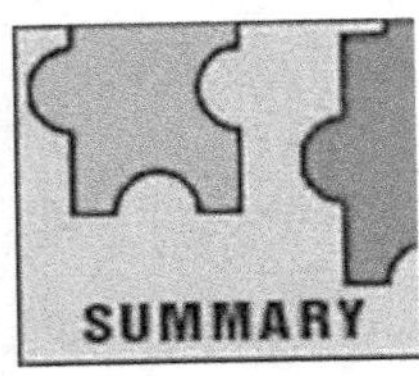

1. Recommended educational requirements to be an iridologist or nutritional consultant include a basic anatomy and physiology course, iridology or nutrition training and work experience in the field.
2. Sources for continuing education include the Internet, magazines, books, journals, research articles and other courses about natural medicine.
3. There are a wide variety of educational resources available for the advanced iridologist or nutritional consultant

Please take the time to answer these questions:

1. What are the recommended educational requirements to be an iridology or nutritional consultant?
2. List and explain sources of information useful for continuing education.
3. List some educational resources available for the advanced iridologist or nutritional consultant?

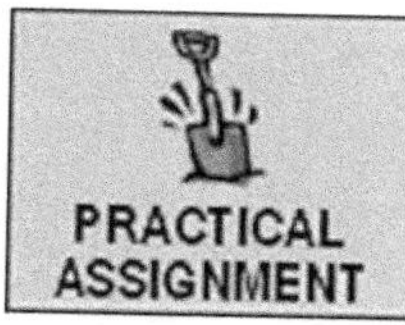

1. Start reading about basic anatomy or physiology or even better take a course.
2. Source some good magazines about health, iridology or nutrition as well as books, journals and Internet sites.

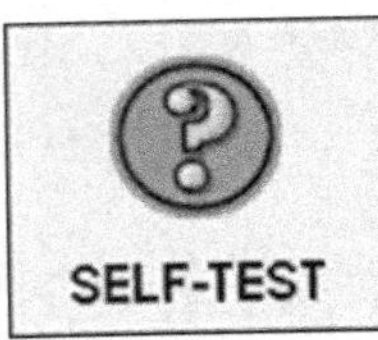

Chapter 9 Self-Test

1. **Basic recommended educational requirements to be an iridologist include:**
   a) Anatomy and physiology
   b) Iridology course
   c) Experience in the field
   d) All of the above

2. **Basic recommended educational requirements to be a nutritional consultant include:**
   a) Anatomy and physiology
   b) Nutrition course
   c) Experience in the field
   d) All of the above

3. **Anatomy and physiology training should include:**
   a) just the body organs
   b) all the body systems, organs and tissues in the body
   c) just human tissues
   d) all of the above

4. **Continuing education includes:**
   a) Reading books
   b) Reading journals and research articles
   c) Taking extra courses
   d) all of the above

5. **Courses that are optional but are useful to the iridologist or nutritional consultant include all except:**
   a) symptomology
   b) holistic medicine
   c) mathematics
   d) diseases

6. **Iridology and nutrition resources for the advanced student include:**
   a) Case studies
   b) Brown-eye iridology
   c) Genetic constitutions
   d) All of the above

7. **Ways to achieve practical experience include:**
   a) sitting in with another iridologist or nutritional consultant
   b) reading about it in a book
   c) practicing on friends and relatives
   d) two of the above

8. **The greatest amount of learning comes from:**
   a) reading books
   b) practical experience
   c) taking courses
   d) surfing on the Internet

9. **Concepts that are useful to be familiar with in relation to human anatomy include:**
   a) Blood pressure
   b) The human cell
   c) Temperature regulation
   d) All of the above

10. **A professional iridologist or nutritional consultant should:**
    a) never stop learning
    b) stop learning when they finish their iridology or nutrition course
    c) read, research and keep up with new information
    d) two of the above

Answers can be found at the end of the book

CHAPTER 10

Essential Advice From Frank Navratil BSc. N.D.

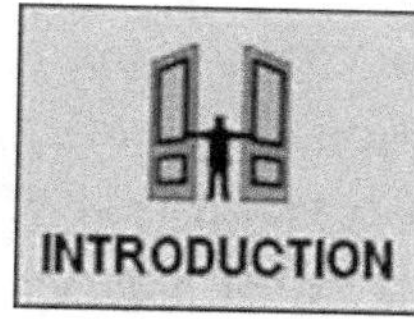

The tenth and last chapter of this book includes advice from Frank Navratil BSc. N.D., world-renowned iridologist, naturopathic doctor and natural health book writer to those wishing to pursue a career in iridology or nutrition.

At the end of this chapter you should be able to:

- Appreciate early humble beginnings
- Understand how honesty, belief and hard work paves the way to success
- Recognize how natural medicine has a promising future
- Learn how to keep motivated and overcome barriers
- Appreciate the importance of caring for yourself to avoid burn-out

- Discover how to find the role and path in life
- Be now equipped to start on the road to establishing their own professional iridology or nutritional consulting practice

Early humble beginnings

When I think to back when I was just starting an iridology and nutritional consulting practice, I remember first using a magnifying lens and light and drawing what I saw in the iris, making notes and then offering recommendations based on what I saw. This method was quite primitive although effective but a good way to start and gain experience in the field. I would have to keep returning back to viewing the iris of my clients and quickly note signs that I saw. I did this for quite a while and had the opportunity to see thousands of irises this way. It was not until a few years later that I began photographing the iris using a 35 mm camera with a circular flash and a long lens. I remember how the flash would almost blind my clients and I would have to take two pictures of each iris (4 in total) to be sure that I got them in focus. Later, I had to develop the film, and usually I found one good iris for each right and left eye out of the four prints that had to be enlarged to a bigger size so I could see the details adequately. The problem with the camera in those days is that I was never completely sure that I took a good picture so once in a while no irises would turn out in focus and I would have to give my patients their money back. I designed an overlay iridology chart that I used over the photos to locate the signs, which took me over an hour to do for each client. I would then manually jot down what I saw and my recommendations. When I first saw a computer assisted iridology software program, I remember I could hardly hold back my excitement. I had been photographing human irises for several years now and had become quite good at it eventually but it had been very time consuming and impractical. Seeing the possibilities of computer software, I decided to invest in an iridology camera; which would be used in combination with this unique software. The result was that I did not need to go and develop film or enlarge prints or take the risk that my photos would not turn out. With digital photography I could retake the photo until I got a clear picture and I could see it all on my computer screen. Not only could I enlarge the image and adjust it for brightness and contrast, but I could overlay a chart precisely over the iris and then automatically scan the iris for color intensity and print out comprehensive reports. This event changed my work so dramatically and allowed me to save so much time and improved the accuracy of my work a thousand fold. My humble beginnings I will never forget and they offered me the opportunity to first get into the field and to learn but with the dawn of computer technology and iridology software, my work in iridology would never again be the same. In recent years I have regularly analyzed over 2000 patients a year and provide them with comprehensive iridology reports and nutritional recommendations. This has also led me to develop my own software, the FYEO PRO- Iridology Scanning, Analysis and Reporting software, which is now being sold all over the world. The moral of this story is that everyone has to start somewhere depending on your finances and time that you have. Whatever humble beginning you have, I sincerely hope that you will also enjoy the success that I have had and gain the priceless rewards from helping so many people.

Follow your heart and your dreams

I once dreamt that I would one day make a difference. That one day I could improve the lives of people. I always believed that if you stay true to what you believe and what is in your heart, you can never lose your way. Many years ago when I was contemplating applying for medical school my mother was struck by cancer and after an 8-year battle, she died. During this time, I began to see how classical allopathic medicine had its limitations and began to study about natural ways to deal with disease. My life would never be the same again. Instead of medical school, I began to study alternative medicine that included iridology, nutritional therapy, Bowen therapy, and other natural therapies. I remember feeling a growing sense of power surging through my body and everything just seemed to make so much sense. I couldn't understand how people had fallen for the primitive health care system based on chemical drug therapy that we have today. I knew at that time my destiny was very clear. My path in life was to learn as much as I can about natural drug-free healing methods, gain experience as a naturopathic doctor and then pass this knowledge on. After years of practicing in Australia and Europe, I did just that. I began to start teaching what I had learned and experienced and began to develop courses that are now being used all over the world. There is still a lot of work to do to educate people on natural cures and after going through this course, you may feel as I do that it is your role to help others so that they can help themselves. There can't be a more satisfying job than helping others. The rewards are immeasurable. Ensure that you are always honest with your clients. If you don't know something, admit it. Don't ever be too proud to refer them to someone else if you are unsure. Stay true to your beliefs, follow your heart and your dreams will come true as well.

Honesty and hard work pave the way to success

I guess I couldn't have chosen a more difficult place to develop iridology than the Czech Republic. Considering a country that had the highest level of intestinal cancer and diabetes in Europe and a very poor knowledge of what even good nutrition was, I had my work cut out for me. At the time that I arrived in the mid-nineties, the communist regime had just recently fallen and the country was living under a new democracy. Alternative medicine had been outlawed for years under the communist regime and even after the fall, alternative medicine was not very well known, and iridology was practically non-existent. When I moved from Australia (a country where alternative medicine was flourishing along with iridology and nutritional therapy) to the Czech Republic, I really did not know whether I could even make a living as a naturopathic doctor. The first couple of years were a very challenging time for me. I began work renting a room from a doctor who was practicing various forms of alternative medicine but was regularly having problems with the ministry of health and would have to justify what he was doing on a regular basis. I remember waiting in that room all week and perhaps I would see two patients. I began to put on presentations at local trade shows that had to do with health and began to write my first article in a Czech health magazine. To my surprise, that article was a dramatic turning point for me and the number of calls I received from patients was staggering. Soon that led to other opportunities to talk in front of groups and to write more about iridology and nutrition in some of the most popular magazines in the country. I was overwhelmed as to the interest that people had and the hunger for natural forms of medicine due to the inadequate state of the health system. Eventually as I continued to write articles and books and to work on my research in iridology and nutrition, my practice grew and grew until I was regularly seeing over 2000 patients a year. People would come from all over the country to visit as well as from neighboring countries as well. After several successful years, I put together the first iridology course to ever be taught in the Czech Republic and was very surprised to get many doctors enrolled as well as lay people. Today after several years of developing one of the first schools of natural medicine in this country, I regularly teach classes of iridology, nutrition, anatomy and physiology, Bowen therapy and other natural medicine courses for the local Czech community as well as seminars around the world. I soon developed a distance education college for international students who come from over 25 countries around the globe. Today doctors, health professionals, naturopaths and healers take my courses around the world and begin or enhance their natural health practices. It has been a long road and a lot of hard work, but I have always tried to build an honest practice and natural health service for my students. When I hear from people around the world how they enjoyed my books or courses, I feel a great sense of satisfaction and a small sense that I can make some sort of difference in the world. Whether you decide to pursue iridology or nutritional counseling, every patient that you see and are able to assist, is in some ways making a difference. I sincerely hope that you will be able to make a difference and together we can change the world, at least partially for the better.

Natural medicine is the future

Our current health care system is not working very well. You can hear about it daily in the papers, on television and in magazines. The quality of health care is not going to get better. Governments do not have enough money to provide quality health care and our population is aging which means more sick people and fewer funds to pay for it. Diseases of our civilization, which include cancer, diabetes, asthma, allergies, arthritis, eczema, digestive disorders, migraine headaches and others, are on the rise. Chemical drug therapy is not the answer to these chronic problems. What are we left with?

Natural medicine is the only way out. Soon, even our doctors and health authorities will work that one out. There won't be enough money to give everyone quality health care so people will have to take care of themselves and work on preventative medicine rather than just waiting until a health problem arises. There will be and already is an increasing demand for natural ways of dealing with disease. People are dissatisfied with their doctors and with the current health system, and it is not going to get any better. They are looking for other options and other alternatives than just popping some pills. People are getting smarter and starting to take more responsibility for their health. They see their parents and don't want to end up in the hospital or on medications all their lives. The quality of life is important to them. There is a growing need and demand for natural non-invasive diagnostic methods such as iridology and as well as nutritional information. Many people have a desire to improve their health but they just do not know where to start. There is so much misinformation on health everywhere you turn, as companies just want to make money. Overnight weight loss programs and diet pills are being sold to millions but unfortunately they don't work and just damage the health of so many people. There is a need for intelligent weight loss programs that include healthy nutritional habits along with exercise programs. An iridology examination can provide so much useful information to patients so that they know what organs and systems have to be strengthened in order to get well. Nutritional counseling along with iridology is one of the best methods I know of to deal effectively with so many diseases that plague our modern civilization. Be assured that if you have decided to pursue a career in iridology or nutritional counseling that you will be a part of the future of medicine.

Reducing barriers

I have mentioned a few of the barriers that I have encountered in my career in natural medicine but here are some others that you will often encounter.

1. Many people will go out of their way to put down or mock natural medicine
2. Many doctors and health professionals will not recognize iridology or natural medicine even though it has been around longer than modern medicine
3. It is very difficult for clients to change diet and lifestyle habits
4. The media is very effective in providing misinformation about health and nutrition
5. There are so many opinions about what is healthy and what is not that it can make your head spin
6. People still often look up to their medical doctors as the only almighty experts on health
7. Clients constantly make the mistake of trying to find a fast acting cure for their health problems and do not have enough patience to care about their long-term health
8. Pharmaceutical organizations, governments and medical associations often do not want to allow natural medicine to grow and will even ban the practice of many effective natural healing methods even though they have proven to cure so many diseases

How do we overcome these barriers? Believe in yourself and in natural means of dealing with disease. It may take a lot of work to convince some people or even some doctors of the benefits of natural medicine but it can be done. Clients have to be educated on the benefits of healthy nutrition and natural drug-free methods of dealing with illness. People have to be educated as to what is really healthy so they do not fall prey to moneymaking advertising schemes. As a professional iridologist or nutritional consultant, you are in a position to teach and educate and to empower those around you. As you gain experience and see how your methods really work, you will have the strength to battle against even those that are against you.

Don't forget yourself

It is common for natural therapists to start a practice, become good at what they are doing and then build a client base that just keeps growing with time. Soon there just does not seem to be any time left as every moment is spent with clients. Don't forget yourself. In order for you to perform quality work, you must be adequately rested and take time out for yourself. Make sure you always give yourself a day or two off a week and have some quality recreation and relaxation time each day. Keep a balance between your work, your personal life, exercise and hobbies.

How to avoid burnout

Sooner or later it is common, especially if you do not pace yourself to suffer from burnout. It is usually a result of working too hard and too long without any break, holiday or quality relaxation time. Feelings of burnout include extreme fatigue, lack of motivation, aggression, boredom and a feeling that you just want to pack it all in. These are all strong indicators that you have been working yourself too hard. Take some time out, reduce your patient load and start doing some of the things that you have been neglecting for so long. Feelings of burnout are telling you that you are not in balance and that something is missing in your life. Maybe you need to spend some more time with family and friends, pursue some hobbies or interests or travel. Give yourself this time to explore what you need and you will once again become refreshed and motivated to go back to work. No one can last forever at such a hectic pace. I know personally a couple years ago when my practice was busting to the limits, I started feeling extremely tired and stopped enjoying my work. It seemed that I just wasn't feeling the satisfaction that I had earlier felt. I decided to take some time out and explore other interests and after a short period of time, my energy levels returned and I felt a lot better. I have learned now to pace myself, reduce my patient load and branch out into other areas that I had been neglecting. You can't live on just work alone!

Your vital role and path in life

This is not really an area that I can advise you on, as I believe that we all have an inherent role or path to follow in our lives and it is up to each one of us to find out what it is. Your life path is your mission in life. I sincerely believe that when you are on the correct path, it brings true happiness, motivation, satisfaction and inner peace. Your intuition is your best source of guidance. For some, their chosen path is found early in life, for others the search takes longer. Keep true to your beliefs and listen to your intuition. It will guide you to your chosen destiny. Have the courage to pursue your dreams. Learn to reevaluate your goals from time to time and ask yourself if you are truly listening within. If you have always dreamt of a career in natural medicine and you feel this strongly in your heart, then go with it. You are not feeling this way for no reason. Something is pushing you forward, possibly to make a change for the better.

My wish to you all

There is nothing that gives me more satisfaction than to see others succeed in their own natural therapy practice. Each one of us is a pioneer when we accomplish this because we are making a change in the world of health. The more of us that can make such a change the greater the chance that one day mankind will view health and medicine completely differently. Perhaps, one day we will learn to respect nature and stop abusing our bodies with drugs and chemicals. Iridology and nutrition are modalities that I strongly believe in and that I know yield positive and long-lasting health benefits.

- I wish you all the greatest success in your endeavors to pursue a career as an iridologist or a nutritional consultant. I believe that they are the future of medicine
- I wish you a smooth ride with as few as possible obstacles or barriers in the way
- I wish you the strength to stay true to your beliefs about natural health and medicine
- I wish you all the satisfaction and rewards in this exciting career
- I wish you many satisfied clients resulting from the work that you will do or are doing
- I wish you lots of luck and a fantastic promising future

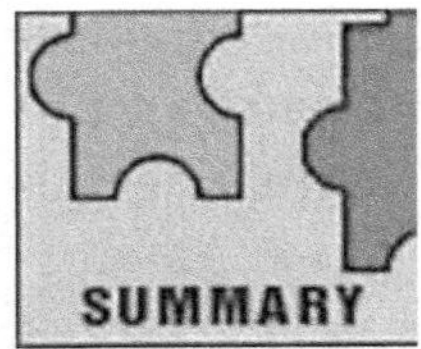

1. Learn to appreciate that it takes a lot of hard work to achieve goals and you often have to start from humble beginnings.
2. Follow your heart and your dreams and you will get on the right path
3. Natural medicine has a very promising and exciting future
4. Often as an iridologist or nutritional consultant you will often come across several barriers
5. As a professional iridologist or nutritional consultant, you are in a position to teach and educate and to empower those around you
6. Ensure that you take time out for yourself in order to reduce the chance of burnout
7. Try to achieve a balance between work, your personal life and hobbies and interests
8. Your life path is your mission in life
9. Being on your correct life path will bring happiness, satisfaction, motivation and inner peace

Please take the time to answer these questions:

1. Why is there a growing need for natural medicine?
2. List some barriers that an iridologist or nutritional consultant may encounter?

3. What is burnout and how can it be avoided?
4. What is meant by life path?
5. What is required to achieve success as an iridologist or nutritional consultant?

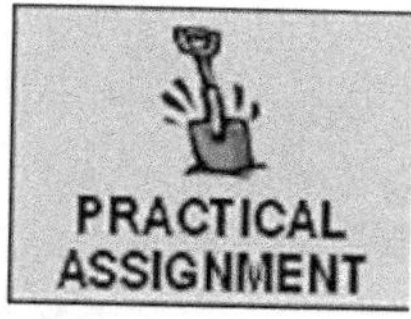

1. Take those first steps in establishing your own business as an iridologist or nutritional consultant
2. Plan your schedule so that it allows for free time and relaxation
3. Set some achievable goals in starting your iridology or nutritional consultation business

Chapter 10 Self-Test

1. **Chronic diseases such as cancer and diabetes are:**
   a) on the rise
   b) decreasing
   c) at the same level they were 10 years ago
   d) none of the above

2. **Burnout is usually caused by:**
   a) too little work
   b) too much work
   c) imbalance
   d) two of the above

3. **Symptoms of burnout often include all except:**
   a) fatigue
   b) lack of motivation
   c) aggression
   d) higher energy levels

4. **Your best source of guidance to get on the correct path in life is listening to (your):**
   a) logic and reason
   b) heart
   c) intuition
   d) two of the above

5. **Your life path is your:**
   a) sequence of experiences
   b) events in life
   c) mission in life
   d) none of the above

6. **It is common for successful natural therapists to:**
   a) suffer from burnout
   b) forget themselves
   c) two of the above
   d) none of the above

7. **Common barriers that can arise include:**
   a) Lack of recognition of natural medicine
   b) Media can provide misinformation
   c) Clients find it hard to make diet and lifestyle changes
   d) all of the above

8. **Overcoming barriers involves all except:**
   a) believing in yourself
   b) educating others
   c) forcing others to comply
   d) inner strength and conviction

9. **Important advice for the successful iridologist or nutritional consultant includes:**
   a) Ensure adequate rest and relaxation
   b) Learn to overcome barriers
   c) Honest, hard work leads to success
   d) All of the above

10. **Starting a successful iridology or nutritional consulting business:**
    a. is hard work that requires honesty, planning and perseverance
    b) requires courage and conviction
    c) brings with it so many priceless rewards
    d) All of the above

Answers can be found at the end of the book

ANSWERS TO MODULE SELF – TESTS

Module 1: 1b, 2b, 3c, 4a, 5d, 6d, 7c, 8d, 9c, 10d

Module 2: 1d, 2d, 3c, 4d, 5b, 6d, 7c, 8d, 9c, 10d

Module 3: 1b, 2d, 3b, 4d, 5d, 6c, 7d, 8d, 9d, 10d

Module 4: 1d, 2c, 3b, 4d, 5d, 6d, 7b, 8a, 9d, 10c

Module 5: 1d, 2d, 3c, 4d, 5d, 6c, 7b, 8d, 9b, 10d

Module 6: 1b, 2d, 3d, 4d, 5d, 6b, 7c, 8a, 9b, 10d

Module 7: 1c, 2d, 3d, 4d, 5b, 6d, 7d, 8c, 9d, 10c

Module 8: 1d, 2c, 3b, 4d, 5d, 6d, 7b, 8c, 9a, 10d

Module 9: 1d, 2d, 3b, 4d, 5c, 6d, 7d, 8b, 9d, 10d

Module 10: 1a, 2b, 3d, 4d, 5c, 6c, 7d, 8c, 9d, 10d

IRIDOLOGY AND NUTRITIONAL BOOKS AND RESOURCES

1. Iridology charts - color laminated by Frank Navratil BSc. N.D.
2. Iridology flashcards - fundamental or advanced sets available
3. Iridology poster of advanced iridology signs
4. Iris Mistr® magnifying lens for Iridology
5. Iridology book "Iridology: For Your Eyes Only" by Frank Navratil BSc. N.D.
6. "Eat Wise by Reading Your Eyes" book by Frank Navratil BSc. N.D.
7. Beginner Iriscope camera with FYEO Basic iridology software
8. Professional Iriscope camera with FYEO PRO iridology software
9. FYEO PRO Iridology analysis, scanning and reporting software
10. "Bowen Therapy" book by Frank Navratil BSc. N.D.

AVAILABLE IRIDOLOGY AND NUTRITION COURSES

IRIDOLOGY

1. "For Your Eyes Only" Iridology home study course - Iris 1 - beginner
2. "For Your Eyes Only" Iridology home study course - Iris 2 - intermediate
3. "For Your Eyes Only" Iridology home study course - Iris 3 - advanced

Also available in the Spanish language

NUTRITION

1. "Eat Wise by Reading Your Eyes" Holistic Nutrition course - Level 1
2. "Eat Wise by Reading Your Eyes " Holistic Nutrition course - Level 2
3. "Eat Wise by Reading Your Eyes" Holistic Nutrition course - Level 3

IRIDOLOGY EDUCATIONAL SOFTWARE RESOURCES

1. "For Your Eyes Only" 100 Iris Case Studies
2. "For Your Eyes Only" Genetic Eye Constitutions (also in Spanish)
3. "For Your Eyes Only" Iris, Pupil and Sclera Signs (also in Spanish)
4. "For Your Eyes Only" The Brown-Eye Iridologist (also in Spanish)

FOR INFORMATION ON ORDERING ANY OF OUR PRODUCTS SEE:

www.irisdiagnosis.org

The world's largest resource of iridology and nutrition education products

Email: irisproducts@irisdiagnosis.org

RETURN TO HEALTH INTERNATIONAL

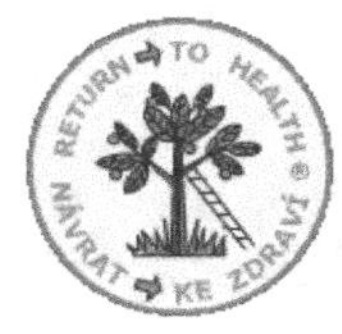

"Welcome to the world of natural medicine"

ABOUT THE AUTHOR

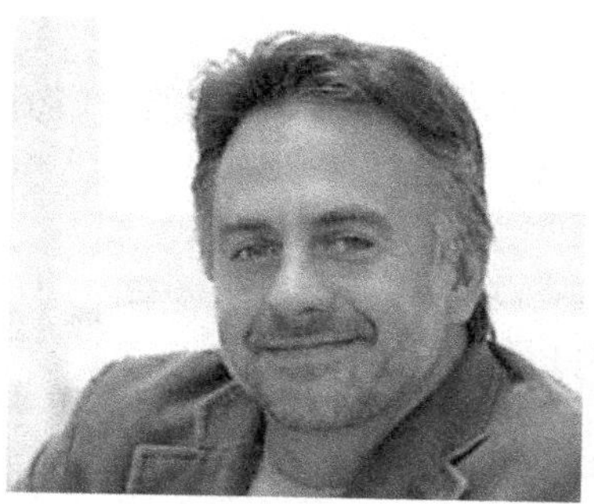

Frank Navratil BSc. N.D. was born of Czech parents in Vancouver, Canada where he completed a degree in physiology and nutrition. In the 1990's he moved to Sydney, Australia where he studied alternative medicine and iridology before practicing as a naturopath, iridologist and nutritionist. Since 1997, he has lived in Prague, the Czech Republic where he has run a natural therapy practice for over 20 years, and directs an international college offering courses in natural medicine.

Frank has given countless lectures around the world on the subject of iridology and Nutrition. He has appeared on several television and radio programs to talk about natural means of diagnosing and dealing with disease. He is the author of the best-selling iridology book, "Iridology: For Your Eyes Only" and the follow-up "Eat Wise by Reading Your Eyes" which have been translated into several languages, as well as "Bowen Therapy."

Based on his clinical research and many years of experience with thousands of patients he has also written and designed the "For Your Eyes Only" series of Iridology courses and "The Eat Wise by Reading Your Eyes" series of Holistic Nutrition courses. These courses have been taken by medical doctors, health practitioners, natural therapists and laypeople the world over.

He has worked, too, in Ethiopia where he studied the effects of malnutrition where he cooperated with an Ethiopian Aid agency to fund the development of an Education Center for the prevention of disease there.

His European naturopathic practice is based on natural holistic methods that allow the body to heal itself. These include iridology, nutrition, vitamin and mineral treatment, Bowen therapy, and diet and lifestyle changes.

CPSIA information can be obtained
at www.ICGtesting.com
Printed in the USA
LVHW090523030619
619950LV00028B/582/P